Chia and Quinoa

Chia and Quinoa

Superfoods for Health

Manju Nehra
Suresh Kumar Gahlawat

CRC Press
Taylor & Francis Group
Boca Raton London New York

CRC Press is an imprint of the
Taylor & Francis Group, an **informa** business

First edition published 2022
by CRC Press
6000 Broken Sound Parkway NW, Suite 300, Boca Raton, FL 33487-2742

and by CRC Press
4 Park Square, Milton Park, Abingdon, Oxon, OX14 4RN

CRC Press is an imprint of Taylor & Francis Group, LLC

ISBN: 9780367529390 (hbk)
ISBN: 9781032214610 (pbk)
ISBN: 9781003080770 (ebk)

DOI: 10.1201/9781003080770

Typeset in Times
by codeMantra

Contents

Preface

Quinoa and chia have gained recognition among consumers worldwide due to their wide variety of nutrients for healthy human life. These crops provide most of the bioactive compounds, gluten-free protein, vitamins, and minerals and are considered an excellent alternative food crop. These crops are extraordinarily adaptable to different agro-ecological zones, highly suited to climate change, harsh environment, and limited availability of resources. Currently, quinoa is expanding in non-native countries, and its cultivation is spreading rapidly due to its very high demand throughout the world. Chia processing results in different coproducts such as noncommercial grains, partially deoiled flour, and rich fiber fraction, among many others. These crops could be reincorporated into the food chain with important technological properties, antioxidant activity included.

The subject matter is presented in this book in a comprehensive and lucid style and intended to provide scientific, authentic, and beneficial information on various aspects of chia and quinoa development in many countries. Moreover, comparative nutritive values, the role of vitamins, minerals, and fatty acids in the human body, products, the role of different processing methods in quinoa and chia, functional properties, and comparative analytical constitutional profile of both the crops are discussed in detail. Thus, this book has enormous scope and opportunities to boost quinoa and chia production, address food and health security problems, increase farm-output, promote food industries and generate employment. It is intended to assist agri-business planners, policy makers, researchers, industrialists, teachers, students, and farmers the world over who are interested in quinoa- and chia-based enterprises for their livelihood. The future is of new alternative crops to cereal and pulses. Quinoa and chia are the new superfoods of the generation and hence show a bright future in the food market.

Acknowledgments

When the whole atmosphere encourages learning, learning is inevitable. We enormously enjoyed writing this book due to our interest in exploring the capabilities within ourselves; we write here today thanking almighty for his immense blessings at all times, which enabled our souls to flourish. The most powerful potential of a human being is when he finds strength in the cosmic topsoil where there are infinite ways to fail. With a project comes enlightenment; we have been enlightened that nothing lasts forever; there is an ordinary way of doing different tasks.

We are indebted to our lessons learned of present and past, our parents, our strength, our life partners, and our children; we appreciate the time they invested in helping us with this project. Our whole-hearted gratitude to Dr. Aruna Sharma and Mrs. Sunita Sangwan, who have been pillars of strength and stood by our side at all times. A special thanks to our spouses, who have played significant roles in completing the project by their constant encouragement. We thank our whole families who prayed for our health during this time and motivated our determination and focus. At some tough times, our light goes out and is rekindled with a spark from another special person; each of us has cause to think with deep gratitude of those who have lit the flame within us.

We are also thankful to the authorities of Chaudhary Devi Lal University, Sirsa, India for constant motivation and encouragement for the entire service period. Last but not the least, we are grateful to the publisher and editorial team for accepting the proposal as well as editing the chapters. We wish to thank all the people who have contributed in completing this venture in one way or another.

About the Authors

Dr. Manju Nehra is Chairperson, Department of Food Science and Technology, Chaudhary Devi Lal University, Sirsa (Haryana, India). Her professional career spans 14 years in which she has been an academician. She completed her BSc in medical stream from Kurukshetra University, Kurukshetra and MSc in Food Technology from Guru Jambheshwar University of Science and Technology, Hisar. Her doctorate degree was also from GJUS&T, Hisar. Her research work was related to the efficacy of natural antioxidants in enhancing the shelf life of oils.

Since 2007, Dr. Nehra has served as a faculty member in the Department of Food Science and Technology, Chaudhary Devi Lal University, Sirsa. She is actively working in new product development from traditional Indian crops, fruits, and vegetables and improving the livelihood of farmers by conducting lectures and workshops on minimal processing and preserving techniques. She has participated in various national and international conferences and presented her research work in lectures and posters. She has published more than 30 research papers in journals of national and international repute. She is actively contributing to university administration by providing services as Director of Youth Welfare. Dr. Nehra has four books to her credit. Her website is a vital public source of information about the changing scenario of human nutrition.

She is associated with various professional bodies such as AFSTI, AMI, and Punjab science congress and provides consultancy services to various agro-based industries. Dr. Nehra is actively involved in curriculum development and nutrition counseling. She has a profound interest in teaching, student counseling, environmental conservation, and traveling, besides hygiene and nutrition.

Dr. Suresh Kumar Gahlawat is a Professor in the Department of Biotechnology as well as Dean of Academic Affairs at Chaudhary Devi Lal University, Sirsa (Haryana, India). He has been presented with various prestigious fellowships and awards from institutes around the globe. He is a renowned scientist and has published more than 100 research papers in national and international reputable journals. Dr. Gahlawat has published more than eight books and has completed many skill enhancement training seminars in universities in India and abroad. The Department of Biotechnology, Government of India, awarded him an overseas associateship to conduct higher research in FRS Marine Laboratory, Aberdeen, UK, from March 30, 2007 to March 07, 2008. He was also awarded by the Department of Science & Technology, GOI in FRS Marine Laboratory, and Aberdeen, the UK, from March 19, 2003 to March 14, 2004. He was awarded Certificate of Commitment by Central Vigilance Commission, Satarkta Bhawan, GPO Complex, INA, New Delhi, upon adopting the Integrity Pledge to uphold the highest standards of honesty and integrity and to follow probity and the rule of law in all walks of life. Dr. Gahlawat has visited many laboratories including Marine Laboratory, Aberdeen, UK: FRS BBSRC, Pirbright, UK (Reference laboratory and working on exotic viruses); CEFAS, Weymouth, UK (Reference laboratory for IPN and SVC viruses); University of Stirling, UK (Working on DNA vaccines, Real-time PCR). Several gene sequences/SNPs have been submitted to GenBank, NCBI, the USA, by Prof. Gahlawat. He has guided many PhD scholars and MSc students and mentored hundreds of students to pursue their careers in academics and industries. He served as chairperson of various departments in the university and held different administrative positions such as Dean of Students Welfare, Dean of Colleges, Dean Faculty, and Dean Research. He is contributing to the science fraternity by motivating young scientists with his enthusiastic approach.

Dr. Gahlawat has completed four R&D projects from UGC, ICAR, and Government of Haryana. His research interests include the development of molecular diagnostic methods for bacterial and viral diseases.

Conflict of Interest

The authors declare no conflict of interest. No one except authors had a role in the study's design, and in the writing of the manuscript, or in the decision to publish the results. Also, the material, data, and research reprinted in the manuscript drafting are duly acknowledged in references. All tables and figures are provided with references from which they are reprinted. There is no intention to copy any material without citing the reference. If found, authors will be responsible for the act (the publisher will not be considered responsible for any act of plagiarism or data copying). The manuscript is duly checked by the software 'Grammarly', and the plagiarism level is below 9% for every chapter (most of the chapters are with 1–3% plagiarism only).

Dr. Manju Nehra
Chairperson, Department of Food Science and Technology,
Chaudhary Devi Lal University,
Sirsa(125055),
Haryana (India)

1 Introduction – Quinoa and Chia

Chenopodium and Salvia are the recent foods of interest to food scientists worldwide because of their excellent nutritional qualities. These pseudocereals are considered new functional foods, and food scientists and nutritionists are showing keen interest in studying the properties of Chenopodium and Salvia.

Being a herbaceous plant, quinoa (*Chenopodium quinoa* Willd.) is a tetraploid and halophytic crop. Quinoa is also considered a part of the Dicotyledoneae class, Chenopodiaceae family, Chenopodium genus, and quinoa species. It is indigenous to South America (from the Andes region).

Quinoa is considered a sacred food in the history of the Inca civilization. However, its role changed during the Spanish colonial period. Many cultural and religious links, including Spaniards, saw it as 'non-Christian' food and replaced it with other cereal grain crops. Production, consumption, and use of quinoa started to decrease in urban communities slowly, but the cultivation of quinoa in the rural/communal areas ('aynoka') remained preserved. Localized cultivation resulted in the development of different localized varieties of quinoa, depending on that specific aynoka. Quinoa (pseudocereals), considered one of the oldest grown crops in the Andean region of America, with approximately 7,000 years of cultivation history, was domesticated and conserved by the great cultures of the Incas and Tiahuanaco (Jacobson et al., 2003). Quinoa is a pseudocereal crop, which is defined as fruits or seeds of nongrass species consumed in a very similar way as cereals with nutritional value competitive to conventional cereal crops, in most cases even better. Fruits of quinoa are achenes, comprising of a single seed enclosed by an outer pericarp (FAO, 2007).

In 1996, FAO cataloged quinoa as a promising crop to solve nutritional problems in human beings due to having high nutritive value and good physical and functional properties. It is considered one of the best vegetable protein sources as its protein profile is much similar to milk proteins and higher than cereal crops such as rice, wheat, and maize. Quinoa seeds can be consumed in various forms. It is used in similar ways as rice, included in soups, puffing is done to make breakfast cereal, or ground to flour to make toasted and baked goods (cookies, bread, biscuits, noodles, flakes, tortillas, pancakes) (Bhargava et al., 2006). The production and consumption of quinoa increased exponentially after 2013. It has gained worldwide growing attention due to its nutritional and functional properties. It can be cultivated under adverse climate conditions and survive extreme environmental stress. The plant quinoa exhibits maximum tolerance to conditions such as drought, frost, and salinity, and it can also grow on marginal soils. These features are significant, considering it as a crop for areas where food insecurity is the issue. Phenotypic flexibility, growth regulation, and activating stress proteins are developed by quinoa that leads to an alteration in plant composition and alterations of natural and social environments. As demand

DOI: 10.1201/9781003080770-1

and production of quinoa in many countries are increasing, native quinoa growing regions are supposed to suffer negative consequences. The cultivation and production of quinoa can go to great lengths in improving food security because of many factors such as its capability to adapt to extreme weather conditions, its low production cost, and above all, its nutritional profile. A nutritious and rich diet may be developed from quinoa which is low in cost, specifically in areas where other nutritious crops are not grown. It may clarify indigenous regions' nutrition, economic, and environmental sustainability and improve food security worldwide.

Although quinoa is an ancient crop, it has attracted consumers' attention as a new food source because of its high protein value and other nutritional properties. Therefore, this book brings an updated review of the chemical composition, physiologically active compounds, and some functional properties of *C. quinoa* that give this outstanding grain potential in human nutrition.

More than 250 species of Chenopodium have been distributed in the whole world. *C. quinoa*, a tetraploid species, is closely related to amaranth and beet varieties originating in the Andean region of Bolivia and Peru. It may be surprising to learn that it has been cultivated in this area for the last 5,000–7,000 years. Quinoa was traded to many ancient cultures such as northern (Venezuela) and southern extremes of South America, namely Argentina and Chile. It is known with different local names in all countries, according to various cultures such as 'supha' in Aymara, 'suba' in Chibcha, 'ayara' in Quechua, 'Dawe' in Mapudungun (southern Chile), or just quinoa or quinua. More than 3,000 varieties are conserved in South American germplasm banks for characterization and conservation. These germplasm banks play an active role in creating possibilities for interchange (informed) of seed materials. Quinoa has been observed to be sown and grown in Asia, North America, Europe, and Africa.

Quinoa is cultivated in rotation with a crop of potatoes which is also a crop of Andean origin. Following this standard practice, quinoa yield is improved, and soil fertility is preserved. It has a cultivation cycle of 8 months in the high Andes, whereas in arid central Chile a short cycle of 4 months is also observed. It has a varied sowing period such as in Altiplano, closer to the Equator (close to 12 hours daylight) it is sown in November whereas it is sown in September to August in the lowlands of more southern latitudes (longer spring and summer days). Maturation and harvest, according to daylength, is done in May in the Altiplano and from February to March in the center south of Chile. Some ecotypes could attain maturity and seed production under irrigation equivalent to only 50 mm of rainfall per season, considered shallow irrigation fall for any crop species. Quinoa seems to have extraordinary, exceptional physiological adaptations for high water usage efficacy under stomatal closure, besides efficient roots for water capture.

The addition of organic matter may increase the yield of grains and water use efficiency in arid areas. Strong tolerance has also been demonstrated for other stressful conditions such as salty soils and cold climates. Quinoa can be grown in various climates, including marginal soils, and under a wide range of soil pH (6.0–8.5). The plant is also not affected by low temperatures even as cold as −1°C. Adding to its unique features, it may tolerate very high temperatures up to 30°C–35°C. Quinoa is considered resistant to cold temperatures even if the frost occurs before flowering. Significant damage may be seen in the plant if frost occurs after the flowering time. Although quinoa is a drought-tolerant crop with low water requirements, the yield is significantly affected by irrigation patterns. Its development can even be seen in regions where the annual rainfall is in the range of 200–400 mm, but it has been proven that it can be grown in southern Chile with yearly precipitation as high as 3,000 mm. Quinoa crop gives a good response in nutritionally poor soils, but it does respond well to nitrogen fertilization, and nitrogen significantly increases seed production and protein content. Being a dicot plant, quinoa is not considered an actual grain, like typical cereal (monocot) grains; it is instead named as fruit and called a pseudocereal and even sometimes a pseudo-oilseed. It has an exceptional balance of fat, oil, and protein. Quinoa can grow from approximately 1–4 m in height. The seeds of quinoa can germinate at a high-speed rate, i.e., in a few hours after being experiencing moisture in the climate. Plant roots can penetrate up to almost a depth of 30 cm if appropriately sown in the soil.

Its stem is cylindrical, 3.5 cm in diameter; it can be either a straight stem or branch. The color of the stem is variably diverse. Depending on the variety, its color changes from white, yellow, or light brown to red. Leaves are shaped like a goose-foot. The flowers of the quinoa plant are incomplete and do not have petals. It has hermaphrodite flowers located at the distal end of a group and female flowers located at the proximal end. Seeds of quinoa are flattened and round, having a diameter from about 1.5–4 mm; the weight of about 350 seeds is around 1 g. The size of the seed is variable, and the color is found from whitish-gray and black, having tones of yellow, rose, red and purple, and violet. There may be very colorful mixes in the same panicle, where black is dominant over red, and yellow turns dominating the white seed color (Figure 1.1).

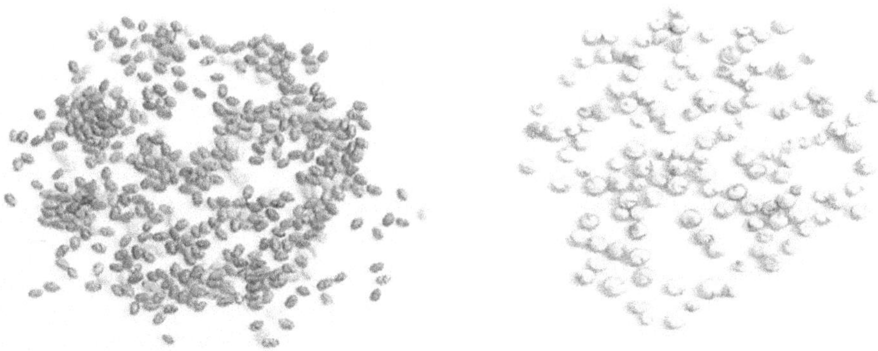

(a) (b)

FIGURE 1.1 Chia seeds (a) and quinoa seeds (b)

The nutritional quality is of quinoa is very impressive. It contains all the major nutrients in proportionate quantity. From quality parameters also, quinoa is known as a substitute for many other crops. The quality of proteins is determined by the proportions of essential amino acids, which are not synthesized by animals and must be provided from outside sources. If only one of these amino acids is limiting, the others will be broken down and excreted, resulting in poor growth of livestock and humans

TABLE 1.1
Essential Amino Acid Profile (g/100 g protein)

Amino Acid	Quinoa (1)	Chia (2)
Histidine	2.9	1.37
Leucine	5.9	4.15
Isoleucine	3.6	2.42
Lysine	5.4	2.99
Methionine + Cysteine	3.6	2.78
Phenylalanine + Tyrosine	6.1	3.88
Threonine	3.0	1.8
Valine	4.2	2.85
Tryptophan	1.2	–
Alanine	4.2	2.68
Glycine	4.9	2.28
Proline	5.5	1.99
Serine	4.0	2.62
Glutamic acid	13.2	24.3
Aspartic acid	8.0	7.29
Arginine	7.7	4.23

References: Amino acid Kozioł, 1992, Dini et al., 2005, Repo-Carrasco et al., 2003, and Gonzalez' et al., 2014. His, histidine; Ile, isoleucine; Leu, leucine; Met + Cys, methionine + cystine; Phe + Tyr, phenylalanine + tyrosine; Thr, threonine; Val, valine; Lys, lysine; Trp, tryptophan. ND, not detected.

and loss of nitrogen in the diet. Ten amino acids are strictly essential: lysine, isoleucine, leucine, phenylalanine, tyrosine, threonine, tryptophan, valine, histidine, and methionine, all of which are present in quinoa (Table 1.1), providing it with a similar value to casein, the protein of milk. Koziol in 1992 showed that protein content in quinoa grain ranges from 13.8% to 16.5%, with an average of 15%. Wright et al. also reported the same pattern of protein content, i.e., 14.9% and 15.6% for sweet and bitter quinoa, respectively, from Bolivia. De Bruin studied the protein content of four genotypes of quinoa, reporting a range of 12.9%–15.1%. According to values indicated by FAO/WHO/UNU, quinoa protein can supply around 180% of the histidine, 274% of the isoleucine, 338% of the lysine, 212% of the methionine + cysteine, 320% of the phenylalanine + tyrosine, 331% of the threonine, 228% of the tryptophan, and 323% of the valine recommended in protein sources for adult nutrition. Also, cysteine and methionine, containing sulfur, are higher concentrations than other plants, probably due to the type of land (volcanic) where this plant originated.

The content of essential amino acids in quinoa is higher than in common cereals. Mahoney et al., working with Bolivian quinoa, concluded that protein contained high amounts of lysine.

Dini et al. (2005), using decorticated quinoa, found that the composition of quinoa is nutritionally comparable or superior to other commonly consumed grains of cereals. When extracted, quinoa proteins' solubility could be improved by enzymatic hydrolysis. Quinoa is also considered one of the best leaf protein concentrate sources and so has excellent capabilities as a protein substitute for food and fodder and in the pharmaceutical industry.

Starch, the principal biopolymeric constituent of plants (grains, seeds, and tubers), occurs typically in granular forms of various shapes and sizes in quinoa. Starch provides the primary source of physiological energy in the human diet, and accordingly, it is classified, in general, as an available carbohydrate. In quinoa, starch is the most crucial carbohydrate in all grains, making up approximately 58.3%–64.5% of the dry matter, according to studies of Repo-Carrasco et al. (2003), of which 11% is amylose. Granules of quinoa starch have a polygonal form with a diameter of 2 μm, being smaller than starch of the common grains.

The petite size of the starch granule can be beneficially exploited by using it as a biodegradable filler in polymer packaging. It can be used as an ideal thickener due to its excellent freeze–thaw stability in frozen foods where resistance to retrogradation is desired. In addition, quinoa flour contains high percentages of D-xylose and maltose and low glucose and fructose contents, which allows its use in malted drink formulations. Also, D-ribose and D-galactose, and maltose content would result in a low fructose glycemic index. RepoCarrasco et al. (2003) reported quinoa 1.70 mg/100 g of glucose, 0.20 mg/100 g of fructose, 2.90 mg/100 g of saccharose, and 1.40 mg/100 g of maltose.

Among minerals, quinoa has a high calcium, magnesium, iron, copper, and zinc content. Many minerals in quinoa are at concentrations more significant than that reported for most grain crops. Provided that they are found in bioavailable forms, calcium, magnesium, and potassium are present in sufficient quantities for a balanced human diet.

For instance, Ruales et al. (1993) and Ahamed et al. (1996) reported in their study that in quinoa, iron, magnesium, calcium, and phosphorus levels are also higher than those of maize and barley: iron was 82 mg/kg, and calcium was found to be 874 mg/kg. Its seeds also have about 0.29% magnesium than 0.17% of wheat and 0.16% of corn. Schlick and Bubenheim, when comparing quinoa from various sources from Peru, Chile, the USA, and Bolivia, reported that the mineral concentrations for quinoa seem to vary drastically. This may occur due to the soil type in the region and mineral composition, and fertilizer application in that specific area. The distribution of minerals within the grain is also a significant concern. Konishi et al. studied this issue, and they used scanning electron microscopy with energy dispersive X-ray detection on quinoa seed (with and without epicarp) and found that minerals like K, P, and Mg were located in the embryo, while Ca and P in the pericarp were associated with pectic compounds of the cell wall. At the same time, sulfur is found to be uniformly distributed in the embryo. The iron has been reported as highly soluble and thus could be readily available to anemic populations.

Vitamins are compounds that are essential for the health of human beings and animals. According to the solubility of vitamins, they are divided into two groups: hydro- and lipo-soluble. Traditionally, vitamins were considered the most widely added chemical agents to enhance the nutritional values of food products. Some vitamins

TABLE 1.2
Chemical Composition of Quinoa and Cereals and Legumes (g/100 g dry wt)

	Fat (g/100 g)	Protein (g/100 g)	Ash (mineral constituents) (g/100 g)	Fiber (g/100 g)	Carbohydrates (g/100 g)	Energy (kcal/100 g)
Quinoa	6.2	16.3	3.9	2.9	69.0	398
Rice	2.3	7.7	3.4	6.3	81.4	373
Barley	1.8	10.9	2.2	4.6	8.9	384
Maize	4.8	10.6	1.7	2.4	82.1	407
Wheat	2.6	15.1	2.2	2.9	77.4	391
Lupin	7.5	39.0	4.0	13.7	35.5	362
Beans	1.4	27.9	4.7	5.2	61.1	366
Soybean	18.7	37.1	5.3	5.7	34.4	450

may also help in lowering the toxic compounds formed in chemical reactions, such as the Maillard reaction (Table 1.2).

The quinoa seeds are rich in α-carotene and niacin. Raules and Nair have also reported in their studies that quinoa contains appreciable amounts of thiamin (0.6 mg/100 g), folic acid (78.1 mg/100 g), and vitamin C (16.4 mg/100 g). Kozioł (1992) compared the vitamin contents of quinoa with some cereals such as rice, barley, and wheat. He reported that quinoa contains substantially more riboflavin (B2), α-tocopherol (vitamin E), and carotene than those cereals. In terms of a 100 g edible portion, quinoa supplies 0.22 mg vitamin B6, 0.63 mg pantothenic acid, 23.5 g folic acid, and 7.1 g biotin. Likewise, Repo-Carrasco et al. (2003) also reported that quinoa is rich in vitamins A, B2, and E. The vitamin E content in quinoa is considered essential as it is a potent antioxidant even at the cell membrane level, protecting the cell membranes against damage caused by free radicals. Quinoa contains lipids oil in the range from 1.7% to 9.6%, with an average of 5.0%–7.2%, higher than that of maize (3%–4%). The human body synthesizes numerous fatty acids known as 'non-essential fatty acids' because they are not essentially needed in the diet. However, because the body cannot produce all the fatty acids, we need to consume a decadent meal in essential fatty acids (EFAs). The EFAs are meant to metabolize the longer-chain fatty acids of 20 and 22 carbon atoms. There are two known EFAs: omega-3 (ω-3) and omega-6 (ω-6). Linoleic acid is metabolized to arachidonic acid and linolenic acid to eicosapentaenoic acid (EPA) and docosahexaenoic acid (DHA). Linoleic acid is among the most prominent polyunsaturated fatty acids in quinoa; polyunsaturated fatty acids have many positive effects on cardiovascular disease and improved insulin sensitivity. The reported total lipid content in quinoa is 14.5% with an unsaturated level of about 70%, having linoleic and oleic acids in percentages of 38.9% and 27.7%, respectively. At the same time, Ahamed et al. reported in another study that quinoa fat had a high content of oleic acid (24%) and linoleic acid (52%). Repo-Carrasco et al. (2003) reported from Peruvian quinoa that the highest percentage of fatty acids is 50.2% for linoleic acid (ω-6) and 4.8% for linolenic acid (ω-3).

Natural antioxidants may play an essential role in inhibiting free radicals and oxidative chain reactions within tissues and membranes. Analysis of antioxidant activities of extracts and fractions is considered an essential step before the isolation of antioxidant phytochemicals they contain as it is a well-known fact that antioxidants are the compounds that can retard or inhibit the oxidation of lipids or other molecules by inhibiting the initiation or propagation of oxidizing chain reactions. When added to foods, antioxidants minimize rancidity, delay the formation of toxic oxidation products, maintain nutritional quality, and increase shelf life. Pasko et al. (2010) showed that pseudocereal seeds and sprouts show relatively high antioxidant activity. Another group of scientists evaluated the antioxidant activity of various extracts from quinoa (Japan) and its relative Amaranthus, finding different values among the samples. In addition, Pasko et al. reported that quinoa presents higher antioxidant activity than amaranth using different methodologies: ferric reducing/antioxidant potential, 2,2-azinobis(3-ethyl benzothiazoline 6-sulfonate) (ABTS), and 2,2-diphenyl-2-picryl-hydrazyl (DPPH). The antioxidant activity of quinoa might be of particular interest to medical researchers and needs further attention regarding its utilization as a potent natural antioxidant.

Several antinutritional substances found in quinoa, such as saponins, phytic acid, tannins, and protease inhibitors, negatively affect the performance and survival of monogastric animals when it is used as the primary dietary energy source. Although saponins are considered the primary antiquality factors associated with quinoa, they also have some interesting biological properties. Saponins are natural detergents made of glycosylated secondary metabolites distributed throughout the plant kingdom; they are a part of a diverse group of compounds characterized by their structure containing a steroidal or triterpenoid aglycone of one or more sugar chains. The quinoa is surrounded by an epicarp that contains saponins showing a characteristic bitter or astringent taste. The saponin concentration can classify quinoa, and their content depends on the quinoa variety: 'sweet' (free from or containing 0.11% of free saponins). Stuardo and San Martin reported that the content of saponins varies in quinoa between 0.1% and 5%. From the nutritional or pharmacological point of view, saponins could also have some value. They can increase membrane permeability, thus increasing food intake at the intestinal level or even for drug assimilation. Other applications include raw materials for the production of hormones and immunological adjuvants. There are also reported to be active ingredients in various natural health products, such as herbal extracts. Stuardo and San Martín, Keukens et al. (1995), and Armah et al. (1999) reported the antifungal activity of quinoa saponins due to their capacity to associate with steroids of fungal membranes. This caused damage to its integrity and pore formation, probably the basis of the novel molluscicide derived from the husks of quinoa, discovered and developed by San Martín et al. Phytic acid usually is present in the outer layers of quinoa, as in the case of rye and wheat, and is also evenly distributed in the endosperm. Phytic acid binds minerals, thereby rendering them unavailable for metabolism. The concentration of protease inhibitors in quinoa seeds is consumed grains and does not pose any serious concerns.

Some Leguminosae, combined with some cereals, might improve proteic profiles of high-quality foods due to amino acid compensation, a good strategy also used with quinoa food for children in the Andean region. Nsimba et al. (2008) used quinoa and amaranth in bread, pasta, and baby foods. Tannins, which are polyphenolic compounds, form complexes with dietary proteins and also with digestive enzymes. In addition to proteins, humans require minerals for their everyday life processes, particularly essential minerals, those necessary to support adequate growth, reproduction, and health throughout the life cycle. Because they cannot be synthesized, minerals are necessarily obtained from the diet, and thus animals require a mineral intake for the long-term maintenance of body mineral reserves.

Minerals are involved in many vital functions in the body, e.g., cofactors of hundreds of enzymatic reactions, bone mineralization, and protection of cells and lipids in biological membranes (antioxidant properties). Low intake or reduced bioavailability of minerals may lead to deficiencies, which causes severe impairment of body functions. Quinoa content is rich in minerals such as calcium, iron, zinc, magnesium, and manganese, which give the grains high value for different target populations. Antioxidant properties conferred by vitamin E and ω-3 fatty acids, plus the neuronal activity of tryptophan amino acid and vitamin B complex, can be powerful aids in brain function. Besides, zinc helps the immunological system, and magnesium is also essential during the formation of neuromessengers and neuron modulators. Quinoa also improves some insulin-like forms, which are active as growth hormones. The low glycemic index makes quinoa suitable for diabetic patients (low fructose and glucose). As mentioned by Oshodi et al. (1999) in earlier years, celiac and lactose-intolerant subjects should also be quinoa consumers because of their gluten-free nature and their rich protein levels, similar to milk casein quality.

The quinoa seeds from different origins, including long-distance regions of Chile, show different isoflavone concentrations, particularly daidzein and genistein. These hormones are implicated in plant physiology (protection from pathogens, UV light, and nitrogen-limited soils) and could be recognized by alpha and beta receptors of estrogens in humans. These endoplasmic reticulum-linked receptors are implicated as inhibitors of tyrosine kinase enzymes and as antagonists of vessel contraction. They also reduce arterial resistance, benefit bone density, and stimulate osteoprotegerin secretion by osteoblasts, in addition to its antioxidant properties.

Researchers have studied the physicochemical, nutritional, and functional properties of quinoa. From ancient and historical data to current laboratory scientific evidence, quinoa was cultivated for its nutritional value. After being abandoned in favor of old-world crops, it is now starting to be rediscovered by modern scientific approaches. While probably giving slower speed to quinoa recovery, Bitter seed coat saponins might now be helpful for its 'take-off' among farmers for a broader range of consumers, as such saponins also have important agropharmacological and cosmetic industrial uses. From the point of view of vegetarian consumers, quinoa, in combination with other cereals, might easily replace meat with a great future in modern, conscient, and more ecological food habits. Functional properties given by vigorously active compounds like minerals, vitamins, fatty acids, and antioxidants make of this small and noble grain a solid contribution to human nutrition, particularly for all cell processes requiring antioxidant protection of membranes, like neuronal activity, with minerals and amino acid contents with potential implications for aiding memory and lowering anxiety under stressful conditions.

CHIA SEEDS

Chia is also considered a superfood crop as quinoa. It is an annual herbaceous plant that is native to southern Mexico and northern Guatemala. It has its unique name from the Latin word 'salvere', referring to the curative properties of the well-known culinary and medicinal herb Salvia officinalis (Dweck, 2005). Nowadays, some species are still used worldwide for their nutritional properties and their beneficial effect on human health. The species *Salvia hispanica* produces numerous dry indehiscent fruits, which are commonly called seeds. The seeds had also been used as a tribute to the capital of the Aztec Empire (Codex Mendoza, 1542) and offered to Aztec gods (de Sahagun, 1579). Due to the religious implications, chia was banned under the rule of the European conquerors and was rediscovered in the 1990s. Since then, it has spread in Argentina, Bolivia, Colombia, Guatemala, Mexico, and Peru and outside America, in Australia, Africa, and Europe (Bochicchio et al., 2015). Chia is a macro thermal short-day flowering plant. This clearly explains that chia seeds are to be sown in late spring and they will not flower until late summer or fall at high latitudes; therefore, the chances of producing seed are low since grain filling is hampered by frost (Ayerza and Coates, 2005).

To ensure an adequate and balanced supply of nutrients to complement the standard diet, consumption of super seeds such as *S. hispanica* L., commonly known as chia seeds, is rapidly increasing. For exploring more about the composition and health benefits of chia seeds, investigations are being carried out. Chia seeds are known as an excellent source of fat (20%–35%), particularly polyunsaturated fatty acids such as α-linolenic (58%–60%) and linoleic (18%–20%) acids. Moreover, high protein levels (16%–25%), mainly prolamins, and dietary fiber contents (23%–40%) have been reported. Vitamins, mostly B complex, and minerals including calcium, magnesium, phosphorus, and potassium have also been found in significant amounts (Table 1.3).

Additionally, the absence of gluten makes these seeds appropriate for celiac patients. Regarding other bioactive compounds, chia seeds are a good source of antioxidants, mainly chlorogenic, caffeic acids, quercetin, and kaempferol. Due to their described composition, chia seeds have been related to different medicinal effects, particularly anti-inflammatory and antidiabetic activities, and positive effects on cardiovascular disease and hypertension.

Chia seeds are currently consumed due to their potential health benefits. The isoflavones present in chia seeds (with average contents of daidzin 0.0066, glycitin 0.0014, genistin 0.0034, glycitein 0.0005, and genistein 0.0051 mg/g of seed) may be used as a new source for the treatment of several disorders. These substances are recognized as anticarcinogenic, with potential therapeutic applications in the prevention of cardiovascular disease. More specifically, phytoestrogens exhibit estrogenic activity and are usually used to treat menopause symptoms, postmenopause, osteoporosis, and other estrogen-related disorders. The high fiber content in chia may convey health benefits because fiber can help increase stool volume and prevent diverticulosis and cancer. Fiber can also help slow the digestion process and the release of glucose, providing antidiabetic effects. Chia had similar effects to fish oil on parameters such as food intake, body weight, thymus weight, thymocyte number,

TABLE 1.3
Chia Nutritional Content

Nutrient	USDA[1]	Jin et al.[2]
Energy	486.0 kcal	562 kcal
Protein	16.5 g/100 g	24.2 g/100 g
Total lipid	30.7	40.2
Ash	4.8	4.77
Carbohydrate	42.1	26.9
Dietary fiber	34.4	30.2
Calcium	631.0 mg/100 g	456 mg/100 g
Iron	7.7	9.18
Magnesium	335.0	449
Phosphorus	860.0	919
Potassium	407.0	726
Sodium	16.0	0.26
Zinc	4.6	6.47
Copper	0.9	1.86
Manganese	2.7	3.79
Vitamin C	1.6	
Thiamine	0.6	
Riboflavin	0.2	
Niacin	8.8	
Vitamin E	0.5	
Folate	49.0 µg/100 g	

[1] USDA National Nutrient Database for Standard Reference, Release 28. 2018. Available online: http: //www.ars.usda.gov/ba/bhnrc/ndl. Accessed 3 May 2019.

[2] Jin, F., Nieman, D. C., Sha, W., Xie, G., Qiu, Y., Jia, W. (2012). Supplementation of milled chia seeds increases plasma ALA and EPA in postmenopausal women. *Plant Foods Hum Nutr*, 67:105–110.

and immunoglobin E levels. The hydrolysis of chia protein creates low molecular weight peptides with antioxidant activities and inhibitory potential of ACE.

The antioxidant potentials of different chia olein fractions were evaluated; the control was 100% milk fat, and the chia olein fractions corresponded to 5%, 10%, 15%, and 20% chia olein completed with milk fat. The values obtained for the control group and the four different fractions were 5.62%, 17.42%, 36.83%, 51.18%, and 74.94%, respectively, evidencing improvements in 2,2-diphenyl-1-picrylhydrazyl free radical scavenging activity. It was suggested that chia seeds could act as an electron donor and scavenger for free radicals because chia protein isolates showed inhibitory effects on angiotensin-converting enzymes that were also far more potent than in *Phaseolus lunatus* L. and *Proteus vulgaris* L. (Fabaceae). Moreover, peptides fractioned from prolamins and globulin were able to participate effectively in the *in vitro* chelation of ferrous ion (Fe^{2+}) in a gastrointestinal tract simulation. Chia also evidenced antiradical activity against 2,2′-azinobis (3-ethylbenzothiazoline

6-sulfonic acid) and 2,2-diphenyl-1-picrylhydrazyl well as angiotensin-converting enzyme activity. The beneficial effects of high contents of bioactive compounds in food products depend on their intake and composition (especially polyphenol compounds, which are directly related to antioxidant properties) and alteration of the contents during digestion. A study evaluated the indices of recovery and bioaccessibility of phenols and flavonoids and their corresponding antioxidant capacity during *in vitro* gastrointestinal digestion of nondefatted and defatted chia seeds. In general, the concentration of polyphenolic compounds increased during digestion; however, only low medium and low percentages of phenols and flavonoids, respectively were available for absorption in the intestinal tract.

Additionally, the presence of high levels of fat appears to impact the bioaccessibility of flavonoids negatively. The divergence of the correlation results obtained between the TPC, TFC, and antioxidant capacity should also be noted. Low bioaccessibility values were obtained for both phenols and flavonoids; however, their potential antioxidant capacity supports the use of nondefatted and defatted chia seeds as food ingredients. Further research is required to describe the stabilities of chia bioactive compounds and improve their bioaccessibility. In terms of *S. hispanica* safety, the UK Committee for Novel Foods and Processes reported potential protein allergenicity by specific IgE binding and immunoblotting. It has been proposed that chia-containing products should carry advisories for consumers with food sensitivities, particularly to sesame and mustard seeds, because cross-reactivity may occur.

Due to its inclusion in dietary supplements, in December 2017, chia seed oil was included in the United States Pharmacopeia; since then, it has been regarded as safe. Chia seed oil is defined as the oil extracted from chia seeds by cold pressing, excluding the extraction methods that include solvent use or external heat. A public quality standard was also established to ensure quality product delivery by manufacturers, and the addition of tocopherols is recommended for oil preservation. The chemical characteristics of chia seed oil were analyzed, and good iodine value, saponification index, and tocopherol content were found. The copper and iron contents were also significant, respectively.

Furthermore, the higher level of polyphenolic compounds than in chia seeds demonstrates its higher antioxidant activity. In terms of its functional properties, the chia coproduct is similar to chia seeds. Apart from decreases in the water holding capacity and gelling capacity, parameters are essential to consider in applications such as producing gelled products cooked meat foods. The low oxidative stability of chia seed oil represents a technological disadvantage. However, it contains natural antioxidant compounds when exposed to environmental factors (light and oxygen), compromising its chemical quality and decreasing its shelf life. Adding additional antioxidants can address the issue. The interest in chia seeds is mainly due to their bioactive composition and nutritional value, which have high potential when incorporated into a balanced diet. These seeds are an essential source of fat (namely polyunsaturated fatty acids, such as α-linolenic and linoleic acids), protein (especially prolamins), carbohydrates, insoluble fiber, vitamins (mainly from B complex), minerals (such as calcium, phosphorus, or potassium), and antioxidants (chlorogenic and caffeic acids, quercetin or kaempferol). Thus, chia seeds and their by-products (such as oil and flour) are increasingly incorporated into different food products. However, more studies are needed to validate their biological effects and confirm the results of scientific investigations to make more conclusive interpretations of the outcomes of chia seed intake and its effects on human health.

BIBLIOGRAPHY

Ahamed, N. T., Singhal, R. S., Kulkarni, P. R., & Pal, R. (1996). Physicochemical and functional properties of Chenopodium quinoa starch. *Carbohydrate Polymers* 31:99–103.

Armah, C. N., Mackie, A. R., Roy, C., Price, K., Osbourn, A. E., Bowyer, P., et al. (1999). The membrane permeabilizing effect of avenacin A-1 involves the reorganization of bilayer cholesterol. *Biophys J* 76:281–290.

Ayerza, R. and Coates, W. (2005). Chia: Rediscovering a Forgotten Crop of the Aztecs. The University of Arizona Press, Tucson.

Ayerza, R. and Coates, W. (2009a). Some quality components of four chia (Salvia hispanica L.) genotypes grown under tropical coastal desert ecosystem conditions. *Asian J Plant Sci* 8:301–307.

Bhargava, A., Shukla, S., and Ohri, D. (2006). Chenopodium quinoa: An Indian perspective. Indus. *Crops Prod* 23(1):73–87.

Bochicchio, R., Philips, T. D., Lovelli, S., Labella, R., Galgano, F., Di Marsico, A., Perniola, M., and Amato, M. (2015). Innovative crop productions for healthy food: The case of chia (Salvia hispanica L.). In: *The Sustainability of Agrofood and Natural Resource Systems in the Mediterranean Basin*. A. Vastola (Ed.), Springer, Berlin, 15–27.

Codex Mendoza. (1542). Edition of Francisco del Paso and Troncoso (1925). Museo Nacional de Arqueologia, Historia y Etnografia, Mexico.

de Sahagun, B. (1579). Historia general de las cosas de Nueva Espan˜a. Reprinted 1982 by School of American Research, Santa Fe.

Dini, I., Tenore, G. C., and Dini, A. (2005). Nutricional amd antinutrional composition of Kancolla seeds: An interesting and underexploited Andine food plant. *Food Chem* 92:125–132.

Dweck, A. C. (2005). The folklore and cosmetic use of various Salvia species. In: *Sage: The Genus Salvia*. S. E. Kintzios (Ed.). Harwood Academic Publishers, Amsterdam, 1–25.

FAO, Food and Agriculture Organization, Ecocrop Database. (2007). Available from: http://ecocrop.fao.org/ecocrop/srv/en/dataSheet?id=2509. Accessed 29 May 2009.

Gonzalez, J. A., Roldan, A., Gallardo, M., Escudero, T., and Prado, F. E. (2014). Quantitative determinations of chemical compounds with nutritional value from Inca crops: Chenopodium quinoa ('quinoa'). *Plant Foods Hum Nutr* 39:331–337.

Jacobson, S. E. 2003. The worldwide potential for quinoa (Chenopodium quinoa Willd.). *Food Rev Int*, 19:167–177.

Jin, F., Nieman, D. C., Sha, W., Xie, G., Qiu, Y., and Jia, W. (2012). Supplementation of milled chia seeds increases plasma ALA and EPA in postmenopausal women. *Plant Foods Hum Nutr* 67:105–110.

Keukens, A. J., De Vrije, T., Van den Boom, C., De Waard, P., Plasman, H. H., Thiel, F., et al. 1995. Molecular basis of glycoalkaloid induced membrane disruption. *Biochem Biophys Acta* 1240:216–228.

Kozioł, M. J. (1992). Chemical composition and nutritional evaluation of quinoa (Chenopodium quinoa Willd.). *J Food Compos Anal* 5(1):35–68.

Nsimba, R. Y., Kikuzaki, H., and Konishi, Y. (2008). Antioxidant activity of various extracts and fractions of Chenopodium quinoa and Amaranthus spp. seeds. *Food Chem* 106(2):760–766.

Oshodi, A. A., Ogungbenle, H. N., and Oladimeji, M. O. (1999). Chemical composition, nutritionally valuable minerals and functional properties of beniseed (Sesamum radiatum), pearl millet (Pennisetum typhoides) and quinoa (Chenopodium quinoa) flours. *Int J Food Sci Nutr* 50:325–331.

Pasko, P., Barton, H., Zagrodzki, P., Izewska, A., Krosniak, M., Gawlik, M., Gawlik, M., and Gorinstein, S. (2010). Effect of diet supplemented with quinoa seeds on oxidative status in plasma and selected tissues of high fructose-fed rats. *Plant Foods Hum Nutr* 65:146–151.

Repo-Carrasco, R., Espinoza, C., and Jacobsen, S. E. (2003). Nutritional value and use of the Andean crops quinoa (Chenopodium quinoa) and kañiwa (Chenopodium pallidicaule). *Food Rev Int* 19:179–189.

Ruales, J. and Nair, B. (1993a). Content of fat, vitamins and minerals in quinoa (Chenopodium quinoa Willd.) seeds. *Food Chem* 48:131–136.

Ruales, J. and Nair, B. (1993b). Saponins, phytic acid, tannins and protease inhibitors in quinoa (Chenopodium quinoa, Willd.) seeds. *Food Chem* 48:137–143.

Ruales, J. and Nair, B. (1994). Properties of starch and dietary fibre in raw and processed quinoa (Chenopodium quinoa Willd). *Plant Foods Hum Nutr* 45:223–246.

Ruales, J., Valencia, S., and Nair, B. (1993). Effect of processing on the physicochemical characteristics of quinoa flour (Chenopodium quinoa, Willd). *Starch/Stärke* 45, 13–19.

Sandoval-Oliveros, M. R. and Paredes-López, O. (2013). Isolation and characterization of proteins from chia seeds (*Salvia hispanica* L.). *J Agric Food Chem*. https://doi.org/10.1021/jf3034978

Stuardo, M. and San Martín, R. (2008). Antifungal properties of 299 quinoa (Chenopodium quinoa Willd.) alkali treated saponins against Botrytis cinerea. *Ind Crops Prod* 27:296–302.

USDA National Nutrient Database for Standard Reference, Release 28. (2018). Available online: http: //www.ars.usda.gov/ba/bhnrc/ndl. Accessed 3 May 2019.

Winkel, T., Flores, R. Á., Bertero, D., Cruz, P., del Castillo, C., Joffre, R., Parada, S. P., and Tonacca, L. S. (2014). Calling for a reappraisal of the impact of quinoa expansion on agricultural sustainability in the Andean highlands. *Idesia* 32:95–100.

Wright, K. H. and Huber, K. C. et al. (2002a). Isolation and characterization of Atriplex hortensis and Sweet Chenopodium quinoa Starches. *Cereal Chem* 79(5):715–719.

Wright, K., Pike, O., Fairbanks, D., and Huber, C. (2002b). Composition of Atriplex hortensis, sweet and bitter Chenopodium quinoa seeds. *J Food Sci* 67(4):1380–383.

2 Physical, Chemical, and Functional Properties of *Chenopodium quinoa*

Quinoa is considered pseudocereals and is a plant with broad leaves that may be used and consumed like cereals. Quinoa was considered an important food crop for the Incas population and remained an essential food for the rural regions of Quechua and Aymara. It was commonly called 'the mother grain' by the Incas; it dates back more than 5,000 years; this native of Andes sustained the Inca community and was considered sacred by the people. Quinoa seed was assumed as the primary crop of the pre-Columbian cultures in Latin America and was consumed as a holy grain. However, after the emergence of the Spaniards, its cultivation and consumption were nearly eliminated and only remained in the traditions of farmers. However, Cusack (1984) discussed the intermittent failure of the green revolution in the Andes and the enormous destruction of other crops by droughts again brought native crops, like quinoa, to the forefront as it showed much less fall in the yields in severe conditions. A quinoa grain possesses an excellent nutritional food quality, and because of that: it is the reason for the tremendous recent interest of food scientists. Quinoa crop belongs to the class Dicotyledoneae, family Chenopodiaceae, genus Chenopodium, and species quinoa. The full name is *Chenopodium quinoa* Willd. (Marticorena and Quezada, 1985) includes the author abbreviation corresponding to Carl Ludwig Willdenow, who discovered the species. The species *C. quinoa* Willd. includes both domesticated and free-living seedy forms (Wilson, 1981, 1988b). Chenopodium species may be used either as whole plants or as parts of the plant. The genus Chenopodium includes about 250 species (Bhargava et al., 2005). It is found at heights of the Bolivian Altiplano at around 4,000 m above sea level. The adaptation of certain quinoa varieties is possible even under marginal environments to produce a high protein and mineral content (Karyotis et al., 2003). Quinoa's aptitude to produce high protein grains under ecologically extreme conditions makes it essential to diversify agriculture in high-altitude regions of the Himalayas and North Indian Plains (Bhargava et al., 2005). Growth of plant, seed quality, seed yield, fresh weight, and dry weight of seeds are influenced by salinity, such as in quinoa. With the increase in salinity, protein content increases in these seeds, whereas total carbohydrate content was decreased (Koyro and Eisa, 2007). While South America is still the largest producer, it is also cultivated in the USA (Colorado and California), China, Europe, India, and Canada and cultivated experimentally in Finland and the UK. Increasing amounts are being exported to the developed world like Europe and the USA. Quinoa is currently produced in Peru, Ecuador, and Bolivia, while all produce of quinoa is exported to Europe and the USA from Chile (FAOSTAT, 2008). Quinoa was first introduced in

DOI: 10.1201/9781003080770-2

TABLE 2.1
Nutritional Composition of Quinoa Seed (g/100 g edible portion)

	Quinoa
Protein	14.1
Fat	6.1
Fiber	7
Carbohydrate	64.2
Ash	2.4
Moisture	13.3
Kcal/100g	368

Source: (USDA, 2018).

England in the 1970s in all European regions, research projects focused on its production for humans and as a fodder crop under temperate conditions (Jacobsen and Stlen, 1993; Jacobsen et al., 1994). Quinoa is an exciting food due to its complete nutritional characteristics. The millennial experience with the quinoa crop allowed ancient populations to recognize the high nutritional value of this food, called by them the 'golden grain', and considered a sacred food (Farro, 2008; Jacobsen et al., 2003). Quinoa seed is rich in nutrients than many other vegetable sources. Its amino acid composition is close to the ideal protein equilibrium recommended by the FAO and similar to milk. Quinoa is found appropriate for the preparation of food products popularly referred to as 'gluten-free' because of the absence of gliadins (gluten-forming proteins present in wheat) and various protein fractions corresponding to gliadins (found in barley, malt, oats, and rye). Moreover, these are the important aspects that enable the supply of more nutritious food and greater variety suitable for patients with celiac disease (Almeida and Sá, 2009; Borges et al., 2010). The anti-nutritional factors present in the quinoa seed are saponins, oxalates, tannins, phytic acid, and trypsin inhibitors, which are present in higher concentrations in the grain's outer layers. Among all these compounds, saponins stand out, which are considered toxic and possess a bitter taste, making its elimination necessary before eating and processing to manufacture food products. Saponin is a natural detergent, soluble in water, which can be easily removed by wet methods (washing with cold water) and dry methods (browning and abrasion) (Mastebroek et al., 2000; Comai et al., 2007; Spehar, 2007; Borges et al., 2010) (Table 2.1).

CARBOHYDRATES

In nature, carbohydrates are among the largest group of natural nutrients, and along with proteins, they form the major components of living organisms. They are the most abundant and economical source of energy for humans. Carbohydrates can be classified according to their degree of polymerization in three main groups: mono, oligo, and polysaccharides (Mahan and Escott-Stump, 2010). Quinoa starch is present between 53% and 68% (dm) in seeds. Dietary fiber has several beneficial effects related to digestibility in the small intestine. Therefore, the high content of quinoa fibers improves the digestibility of food by facilitating the process of absorption of other nutrients present in quinoa in the large intestine (Ogungbenle, 2003). The soluble indigestible fiber content is reported ranging from 1.6% to 6.7% (dm). In quinoa, approximately 3% of simple sugars are primarily present in the form of maltose, followed by D-galactose and D-ribose, plus low levels of fructose and glucose (Abugoch James, 2009). Gluten-free dietary fiber is considered inadequate. Thus, experts recommend a higher intake of whole grains rich in fiber products in the diet of patients with celiac disease (Alvarez-Jubete et al., 2010a).

Starch is considered the main biopolymeric constituent of plants (beans, seeds, roots, and tubers) and is typically found in various shapes and sizes of granules. Quinoa starch granules have a polygonal shape with a diameter of 0.6–2.2 μm, less than the starch of most cereal grains. They may be found as single entities or forming aggregates of spherical or elliptical composite structures. The petite size can be beneficially exploited and used in blends with synthetic polymers to prepare biodegradable packaging. It possesses excellent freeze-thaw stability, which makes it an ideal thickener for sauces, condiments, and soups due to its low gelation temperature and storage stability at low temperatures. Also, in other applications where resistance to retrogradation is desired, it may be used to produce a creamy and smooth texture similar to fats (Lorenz, 1990; Tari et al., 2003; Abugoch James, 2009; Vega-Gálvez et al., 2010). Quinoa starch has an average molar weight of 11.3×106 g/mol, mass lower than waxy maize starch (17.4×106 g/mol) or rice (0.52–1.96×108 g/mol) and more prominent than wheat starch (5.5×106 g/mol), as observed by Park et al. (2007) and Praznik et al. (1999). Quinoa starch has a highly branched structure, with a minimum degree of polymerization of 4,600 glucose units, maximum of 161,000, and a weighted average of 70,000 (Praznik et al., 1999). However, the length of the chain depends on the botanical source, ranging from 500 to 6,000 glucose units.

James Abugoch, in the year 2009, confirmed the findings of Kozioł (1992), stating that the amylose content of quinoa starch ranges from 3% to 23%. The amylose content of quinoa is lower than wheat or maize, more remarkable than some barley varieties, and similar to certain rice varieties. Also, according to Tang et al. (2002), the starchy fraction of quinoa has an average degree of polymerization of 930, much lower than that of barley, which is 1,660.

Carbohydrates in quinoa can be considered as nutraceutical food components because they have beneficial hypoglycemic effects and reduce free fatty acids (details in Chapter 5).

PROTEINS

Proteins participate in constructing and maintaining tissues, forming enzymes, hormones and antibodies, power supply, and metabolic processes. In addition to nitrogen, amino acids provide sulfur compounds to the body. Lipoproteins transport triglycerides, cholesterol, phospholipids, and fat-soluble vitamins (Ahmed et al., 1998b). For some populations globally, including high-quality protein in their diets is a problem, especially for people who rarely consume animal protein and should get them from cereals, legumes, and other grains. Even though the contribution of proteins by these foods is enhanced, insufficient concentrations of some essential amino acids can increase the prevalence of malnutrition (Mujica et al., 2001; Alves et al., 2008).

The nutritional value of a food is measured mainly by its protein quality and digestibility of proteins, which depends on the composition of essential amino acids, and the biological utilization of the amino acids (bioavailability), the influence of present antinutritional factors. Quinoa has a high protein content and an adequate amino acid composition, along with a high concentration of tryptophan.

The proportion of essential amino acids determines the nutritional quality of the proteins, namely those that cannot be synthesized by animals, therefore, must be supplied in the diet. If only one of the essential amino acids is limiting, the others will also not be fully absorbed, resulting in loss of dietary protein and retarded growth. Nine amino acids are considered as essential for human beings: phenylalanine, isoleucine, leucine, lysine, methionine, threonine, tryptophan, valine, and histidine (essential in childhood) as reported by World Health Organization (WHO) in the year 2007, and they all are present in quinoa, providing a protein value similar to casein from milk (Vega-Gálvez et al., 2010). Having an excellent amino acidic balance, being rich in sulfur amino acids and lysine, quinoa can be considered a high-quality protein, unlike the protein content of cereals, which are significantly deficient in lysine (Mujica et al., 2001; Alves et al., 2008).

In 1992, Kozioł was among the scientists who worked a lot on the physical and nutritional properties of quinoa. He stated that the protein content in quinoa grain ranges from 13.8% to 16.5%, with an average of 15% dm. The total protein content of quinoa is much higher than that for barley (11.01% dm), rice (8.79% dm), corn (10.15% dm), rye (dm 11.60%), and sorghum (12.14% dm), getting close to wheat (14.8% dm) (Kozioł, 1992; Comai et al., 2007; Jancurová et al., 2009). Albumins (2S) and globulins (11S) make up most of the storage proteins from quinoa grain (35% and 37%, respectively), while the prolamins are present in low concentrations, and this ratio is variable in different species (Brinegar and Goudan, 1993; Brinegar et al., 1996; Abugoch James, 2009).

LIPIDS

Quinoa is considered an alternative oilseed crop due to its lipidic fraction (Kozioł, 1993). Besides their proteins' high content and good biological quality, quinoa seeds have a much interesting lipid composition of about 1.8%–9.5% (Kozioł, 1993; Masson and Mella, 1985; Ryan et al., 2007; USDA, 2005; Wood et al., 1993). Polyunsaturated fatty acids have gained importance in recent decades due to their health benefits, such as positive effects on cardiovascular disease, metabolism of prostaglandins, and increased insulin sensitivity. Essential fatty acids are essential acids, like linoleic and linolenic acids, necessary substrates in animal metabolism. Quinoa has a fat content between 2.0% and 9.5%, is rich in essential fatty acids like linoleic and α-linolenic, and contains high concentrations of antioxidants like α and γ tocopherol. It has an oil content of around 7% (dm), higher than corn (4.7% dm) and other cereals, and lower than soybeans (19.0% dm). Quinoa has oil content (7% dry basis) higher than corn (4.9% dry basis) and lowers than soy (20.9% dry basis) (Kozioł, 1993; USDA,

2005). Some researchers have characterized the fatty acid composition of quinoa lipids as follows: total saturated 19–12.3%, mainly palmitic acid; total monounsaturated 25%–28.7%, mainly oleic acid, and total polyunsaturated 58.3% – chiefly linoleic acid (about 90%) (Masson and Mella, 1985; Oshodi et al., 1999; Ranhotra et al., 1993; Ryan et al., 2007; USDA, 2005; Wood et al., 1993). Linoleic acid is basically metabolized to arachidonic acid and linolenic acid to Eicosapentaenoic Acid (EPA) and Docosahexaenoic Acid (DHA). EPA and DHA play essential roles in prostaglandin metabolism, thrombosis and atherosclerosis, immunology and inflammation, and membrane function (Simopoulos, 1991; Youdim et al., 2000).

The oil fraction of quinoa seeds has a high degree of unsaturation, with a polyunsaturation index of 3.8–4.6, which makes it highly nutritious. In this fraction, not only the fatty acid composition is essential, another essential characteristic is the presence of a good amount of vitamin E naturally (a-tocopherol), 0.61–2.6 mg/100 g in the seeds (Coulter and Lorenz, 1990; Ryan et al., 2007; USDA, 2005), which acts as a natural defense against lipid oxidation (Ng et al., 2007). This could lead to very stable oil from quinoa seeds, with vitamin E as a natural antioxidant. The (b þ g)-tocopherol content in whole quinoa flour has been reported as 3.4–5.8 mg/100 g (Ruales and Nair, 1993a; Ryan et al., 2007).

PHYTOSTEROLS

Phytosterols have different biological effects such as anti-inflammatory, antioxidative, and anticarcinogenic activity, and cholesterol-lowering capacity, as reported by Moreau et al. in 2002. The levels of phytosterols from QS reported by Ryan et al. (2007) were b-sitosterol 63.8 mg/100 g, campesterol 15.7 mg/100 g, and stigmasterols 3.2 mg/100 g, which are the most abundant plant sterols. These phytosterol levels are higher than in pumpkin seeds, barley, and maize but lower than in lentils, chickpeas, or sesame seeds (Ryan et al., 2007). The recommended doses of free phytosterols are 0.8–1.0 g of equivalents per day, including natural sources. They are essential dietary components for lowering low-density lipoprotein (LDL) cholesterol and maintaining good heart health (Berger et al., 2004).

VITAMINS AND MINERALS

Quinoa is also rich in micronutrients such as vitamins and minerals. Vitamins are compounds essential for the health of humans and animals. Some compounds belonging to the class of sterols and carotenoids can be processed in vitamins in the human body, which is why such substances are termed ‘provitamins’.

Minerals are inorganic and cannot be produced by living beings. They hold a significant role in performing various functions in the body. Lower intake or reduction of bioavailability may generate imbalances in health and impairment of vital functions. The best known are calcium, iron, sodium, phosphorus, potassium, sulfur, magnesium, zinc, copper, selenium, and chromium. These micronutrients must be ingested through well-balanced diet to supply the daily needs. Particular attention should be given to the correct food combinations, preparation techniques, and nutrients to enhance their bioavailability (Cozolino, 2009; Vega-Gálvez et al., 2010).

Potassium is the most abundant mineral found in quinoa grain, followed by magnesium and phosphorus, while iron showed the lowest value (Ogungbenle, 2003). In a study, Ando et al. (2002) and Konish et al. (2004) analyzed that the mineral content in the quinoa grain is getting the highest levels of calcium, phosphorus, iron, potassium, magnesium, and zinc among the minerals analyzed. Some studies show that the quinoa grain shows significantly higher amounts for these minerals when compared to most cereals traditionally consumed in Brazil (Borges et al., 2003; Repo-Carrasco et al., 2003; Bhargava et al., 2006; NEPA, 2011).

The bioavailability of iron present in quinoa may be affected to some extent by saponins and phytic acid present in the seeds. Ruales and Nair (1993a) reported that the amount of phytic acid after the washing process used for the removal of saponins remained high, about 8 mg/g. The procedure for cleaning and washing with water used to remove saponins appears to influence the content of minerals. A significant reduction of 46% in the potassium content, 28% in iron, 27% in manganese, and 8% in magnesium (Rules and Nair, 1993a) was observed. However, as cited by Kozioł (1992) and Rules and Nair (1993a), feeding experiments with animals have shown that iron availability from diets based on quinoa was at least as good as iron availability from ferrous sulfate.

POLYPHENOLIC COMPOUNDS

Pseudocereals may contribute to cardiovascular protection when coronary heart diseases are becoming the leading cause of death in most developed countries and are overgrowing in developing countries. It has been shown that foods rich in dietary fibers are often an important source of vitamins, minerals, phytochemicals, natural antioxidants, and other micronutrients. Cereals and pseudocereals play an important role in providing antioxidants (Gorinstein et al., 2008). Natural antioxidants can play an important role in inhibiting free radicals and oxidation chain reactions within tissues, in particular for the protection of cell membranes, with proven success in neural functions, reducing the risk of degenerative diseases which are associated with oxidative stress such as cancer, cardiovascular disease, and osteoporosis (Nsimba et al., 2008; Alvarez-Jubete et al., 2010b; Vega-Gálvez et al., 2010). Antioxidants are compounds that can retard or inhibit the oxidation of lipids or any other component by inhibiting the initiation or propagation of oxidation chain reactions. When added to foods, antioxidants minimize rancidity, retard the formation of toxic oxidation products, maintain nutritional quality and increase the shelf life (Vega-Gálvez et al., 2010). Quinoa seeds are also a rich source of flavonoids named quercetin and kaempferol glycosides. Zhu et al. (2001) isolated six flavonols glycosylated from quinoa seeds. They found that the two quercetin 3-glycosides showed the highest antioxidant activity than the four kaempferol 3-glucosides present, suggesting that quinoa could represent an important source of free radical inhibition. Quinoa seeds from Japan were found to have the highest antioxidant effect compared to those in South America and other grains, except buckwheat (Hirose et al., 2010). The results suggest that quinoa seeds cultivated in Japan have phenolic compounds, particularly quercetin glycosides, in larger quantities, responsible for their high antioxidant capacity.

ANTINUTRITIONAL FACTORS

Plant sources are not always good for the problems arising because of some compounds derived from secondary plant metabolism. The term 'antinutritional factor' describes the class of compounds present in a wide variety of plant foods, which, when consumed, reduce their nutritional value, interfering with their digestibility, absorption, or utilization of nutrients, possibly causing harmful effects to health if ingested in high concentrations. Therefore, it is crucial to understand the antinutritional factors of conventional and unconventional plants to determine which compounds interfere with their nutritional value (Lopes et al., 2009; Benevides et al., 2011). Different types of antinutritional factors have been identified in different fruits and vegetables. In quinoa seeds, the identified antinutritional factors are saponins, tannins, nitrates, phytic acid, oxalates, and trypsin inhibitors. These antinutrients are present in higher concentrations in the outer layers of the seed. Studies on the possible antinutrients in quinoa are little/scarce, and less is known about its antinutritional or toxic effects that might compromise its nutritional quality in order to incorporate it effectively in the human diet (Santos, 2006; Lopes et al., 2009; Borges et al., 2010). Despite the presence of antinutritional factors in the quinoa grain, these substances can be inactivated or reduced to safe health levels when appropriate techniques for industrial processing or household preparation of this food are used (Borges et al., 2010).

SAPONINS

The quinoa grain has a naturally bitter coating called saponin. Substances found in plants, particularly of the Leguminosae family, are triterpenoid glycosides without well-defined chemical formula; however, in general, we can suggest the following basic chemical formula: CnH2n-8O10 ($n \geq 5$). Four main structures of sapogenins were identified in quinoa: oleanolic acid, hederagenin, phytolaccagenic acid, and 30-O-methyl-espergulagenate (Dini et al., 2001, Zhu et al., 2002, Souza et al., 2004; Farro, 2008). Although they are highly toxic to cold-blooded animals, their oral toxicity in mammals is low, not exerting any adverse effect on the nutritional quality of the protein. Some of the saponins form complexes with iron and zinc, reducing their absorption, but there is no evidence of the formation of complexes with vitamins A, E, and D3 (Gonzáles et al., 1989; Kozioł, 1990, 1992; Rules and Nair, 1993b; Dini et al., 2001; Farro, 2008; Jancurová et al., 2009). Saponins are considered toxic, and due to that, their insecticide, fungicide, and antibiotic properties are also recognized. They present pharmacological potential by modifying the permeability of the small intestine, which may aid in the absorption of specific drugs and reduce the plasma or serum cholesterol by fecal secretion of bile acid and neutral steroids. The pharmaceutical industry is used as precursors to synthesize steroids, hormones, contraceptives, anti-inflammatories, expectorants, and diuretics (Dini et al., 2001; Farro, 2008; Veja-Gálvez et al., 2010). The content of saponins is more significant in the pericarp, accounting for 86% of the total present in the grain, showing that peeling can remove most of this substance. The amount of saponins in the quinoa grain is much smaller than that found in soybeans and other legumes (Chauhan et al., 1992;

Mastebroek et al., 2000; Ando et al., 2002; Abugoch James, 2009). Due to its characteristic bitter taste, the amount of this substance is usually reduced or removed from the outside of the grain to provide better sensory quality and consumer acceptance. Removal is accomplished through a process of selection of sweet varieties or wet methods including washing in cold alkaline water and dry methods including heat treatment, extrusion, roasting, or mechanical abrasion), or a combination of both methods (Koziол, 1990, Dini et al., 2001; Brady et al., 2007; Comai et al., 2007, Spehar, 2007; Farro, 2008; Jancurová et al., 2009). The wet method is the most used household level, and it and can also be used on a commercial scale. However, it has economic and ecological inconveniences due to the large water consumption and the need for drying the grains after washing, besides the contamination of water with saponins waste (Rütte, 1990).

PHYTIC ACID

The bioavailability of components like starch, protein, enzymes, and minerals such as calcium, iron, magnesium, zinc, and copper is compromised due to a highly negatively charged compound-phytic acid, which has also been regarded as a component of antinutritional action. Phytic acid is mainly found in the peel of most cereals and legumes, in concentrations of 1%–3% dry matter, constituting the central phosphate reserve of these seeds. It can also be found in some fruits and vegetables (Ruales and Nair, 1993b; Oliveira et al., 2003; Jancurová et al., 2009). Phytic acid is not only present in the quinoa grain's outer layers, such as in wheat and rye, but it is also distributed uniformly in the endosperm. While phytic acid in quinoa is higher than in grains, no adverse effects were observed in incorporating calcium or iron absorption in bones (Koziоł, 1992). In removing saponins from quinoa seeds by brushing and rinsing, a significant reduction of approximately 30% in the amount of phytic acid also occurs. The concentration of phytic acid in nonprocessed quinoa seed was 10.4 mg/g, while in processed seeds, it was 7.8 mg/g compared with values obtained in whole flour grain, such as rye (7.7 mg/g), wheat (8.7 mg/g), lentils (8.4 mg/g) and faba bean (8.0 mg/g) (Rules and Nair, 1993b). Phytic acid content can be significantly reduced by processes such as steeping, germination, and fermentation. The efficiency related to degradation is higher in processes that promote the activation of phytase, such as fermentation and cooking (Rules and Nair, 1993b; Oliveira et al., 2003; Khattab and Arntfield, 2009).

TANNINS

Tannins are also present in tiny quinoa seeds (0.53%), considerably lower than in rice grains (1.3%), and further reduced after cleaning and rinsing with water. The tannins were higher in peeling (0.92%) compared with bran or flour. However, the bran still contained 46–50% of the total tannin of seeds (Chauhan et al., 1992; Jancurová et al., 2009). Results suggest that the fair use of washing and preparation steps (cooking) of quinoa grain may reduce the harmful effects of tannins, thus improving the digestibility (Borges et al., 2010). In human nutrition, tannin-like antinutritional factors have little consequence because they are thermolabile and are generally destroyed in the ordinary conditions of domestic or industrial food preparation (Khattab and Arntfield, 2009; Lopes et al., 2009). According to Ando et al. (2002), phytates and trypsin inhibitors were higher in the embryo of quinoa seeds. The embryo contained 60% of the total phytate and 89% of the trypsin inhibitory activity compared to the whole grain.

NITRATES

Nitrates are present in almost all plants, and they are essential sources of nitrogen for average growth. High nitrates are found in leaves, especially in the mesophyll, but petioles and stems are the locations of maximum accumulation. Moreover, reproductive organs, fruits, and seeds are supplied with amino acids via the phloem, thus having low nitrate levels. The nitrate present in vegetables may originate in used fertilizers or may be formed on the substrate by nitrification or mineralization (Beninni et al., 2002; Santos, 2006). The levels of nitrate (NO_3) found by Lopes et al. (2009) in quinoa wholemeal 'BRS Piabiru' (63.26 mg/100 g) were twice lower than those reported in vegetables such as spinach, lettuce, radishes, and beets, whose values are presented above 100 mg/100 g of the fresh produce, proving that quinoa offers no disadvantage to diet and health. According to Benevides et al. (2011), the acceptable daily intake (ADI) recommended by the WHO of nitrate ions and nitrite is 3.7 and 0.06 mg/kg of the body weight, respectively. Therefore, for a 60 kg adult, nitrate intake should not exceed 222 mg/day and nitrite 3.6 mg/day, which corresponds to the consumption of 351 g of quinoa wholemeal 'BRS Piabiru'. Thus, according to Lopes et al. (2009), the amount of customarily consumed flour would not endanger consumers' safety.

OXALATES

Oxalate is a toxic substance often found in spinach, beets, chard, rhubarb, tomatoes, nuts, and cocoa. It cannot be metabolized by the human being and is generally excreted through the urine. The absorption of minerals and trace elements is highly influenced by high intake of oxalate, which plays a crucial role in hyperoxaluria; a risk factor for the formation of calcium oxalate stones in the kidneys, due to the ability of the oxalate to form insoluble complexes with divalent cations in the gastrointestinal tract (Santos, 2006; Jancurová et al., 2009; Lopes et al., 2009). Trace amounts of oxalates are present in quinoa seeds, which seems to cause no harm to human health, but studies still need to be conducted as scarce literature is available about this. Saponins are steroid or triterpenoid glycosides, with the latter found more commonly in crops (Francis et al., 2002). These compounds have a bitter taste and are considered toxic in large amounts. They are present in the whole quinoa plant, where their natural function is to defend the plant from the external medium. In general, quinoa seeds contain saponins in the seed coat (except sweet varieties, without saponin or containing less than 0.13%).

Brady et al. (2007) have reported that the bitter taste imparted by saponins and other antinutrients could potentially be reduced by extrusion and roasting processes. Saponins are compounds that contain sugar chains and a triterpenoid aglycone (sapogenin) in their structure (Sparg et al., 2004). Four main structures of sapogenins have been identified in quinoa: oleanolic acid, hederagenin, phytolaccagenic acid, and 30-o-methyl spergulagenat (Zhu et al., 2002). The significant carbohydrates are glucose, arabinose, and galactose. Besides, 20 triterpene saponins have been isolated from different parts of *C. quinoa* (flowers, fruits, seed coats, and seeds) (Kuljanabhagavad et al., 2008; Zhu et al., 2002). Saponins have been considered toxic for different organisms. Meyer et al. (1990) found toxicity to brine shrimp. Woldemichael and Wink (2001) found monodesmoside saponins hemolytically active. The hemolysis may be produced by the interaction of the saponins with membranes, producing pores that lead to rupture of the (Seeman et al., 1973). Kuljanabhagavad et al. (2008) described mainly saponins with an aldehyde group as cytotoxic in HeLa (cervix adenocarcinoma) cell line. Saponins have shown insecticidal, antibiotic, fungicidal, and pharmacologic activity. Woldemichael and Wink (2001) found five quinoa saponins (glycosides of oleanolic acid and hederagenin) that showed some antifungal activity on Candida albicans; Stuardo and San Martín (2008) found higher antifungal activity against Botrytis cinerea with alkali-treated quinoa saponin. Nowadays, saponins have been studied because different beneficial properties to health have been described. Saponins possess a wide variety of biological effects: analgesic, anti-inflammatory, antimicrobial, antioxidant, antiviral, and cytotoxic activity, affecting the absorption of minerals and vitamins and animal growth. They also have hemolytic and immunostimulatory effects, increased permeability of the intestinal mucosa neuroprotective action, and reduction of fat absorption (Güçlü-Üstündag and Mazza, 2007). However, the biological properties of quinoa saponins require further study.

Despite quinoa grains showing some antinutritional factors, it can be concluded that it is a promising crop because these antinutritional components can easily be removed during the manufacturing process or by appropriate handling techniques. Therefore, quinoa has a high nutritional value and has recently been used as a novel functional food because of all these properties.

BIBLIOGRAPHY

AACC. (1990). Approved methods of the American Association of Cereal Chemists. 9th ed., Method 86-06, 1995; II: 1–8. 4. AOAC. Official method of analysis. Association of Official Analytical Chemists. 15th ed., Washington, DC.

Abugoch James, L. E. (2009). Quinoa (Chenopodium quinoa Willd.): composition, chemistry, nutritional, and functional properties. *Adv Food Nutr Res* 58:1–31.

Ahamed, T., Singhal, R., Kulkarni, P., and Pal, M. (1998b). A lesser-known grain, Chenopodium quinoa: Review of the chemical composition of its edible parts. The United Nations University. *Food Nutr Bull* 19:61–70.

Almeida, S. G. and Sá, W. A. C. (2009). Amaranto (Amaranthus ssp) e quinoa (Chenopodium Quinoa) alimentos alternativos para doentes celíacos. *Ensaios e Ciência: C. Biológicas Agrárias e da Saúde* XIII(1):77–92.

Alvarez-Jubete, L. et al. (2010a). Nutritive value of pseudocereals and their increasing use as functional gluten-free ingredients. *Trends Food Sci Technol* 21(2):106–113.

Alvarez-Jubete, L., Wijngaard, H.H., Arendt, E.K., and Gallagher, E, (2010b). Polyphenol composition and in vitro antioxidant activity of amaranth, quinoa and buckwheat as affected by sprouting and bread baking. *Food Chem* 119:770–778.

Alves, L. F., Rocha, M. S., and Gomes, C. C. F. (2008). Avaliação da qualidade proteica da Quinua Real (Chenopodium quinoa Willd) através de métodos biológicos. *E-scientia* 1(1):16.

Ando, H., Chen, Y., Tang, H., Shimizu, M., Watanabe, K., and Miysunaga, T. (2002). Food components in fractions of quinoa seed. *Food Sci Technol Res* 8(1):80–84.

Benevides, C. M. J., Souza, M. V., Souza, R. D. B., and Lopes, M. V. (2011). Fatores antinutricionais em alimentos: Revisão. *Segurança Alimentar e Nutricional* 18(2):67–79.

Beninni, E. R. Y., Takahashi, H. W., Neves, C. S. V. J. and Fonseca, I. C. B. (2002). Teor de nitrato em alface cultivada em sistemas hidropônico e convencional. Hort Brasileira 20(2):183–186.

Berger, A., Jones, P., and Abumweis, S. (2004). Plant sterols: Factors affecting their efficacy and safety as functional food ingredients. *Lipids Health Dis* 3:5.

Bhargava, A., Rana, T., Shukla, S., and Ohri, D. (2005). Seed protein electrophoresis of some cultivated and wild species of Chenopodium. *Biol Plan* 49(4):505–511.

Bhargava, A., Shukla, S., and Ohri, D. (2005). A Karyotypic studies on some cultivated and wild species of Chenopodium (Chenopodiaceae). *Gen Res Crop Evol.*

Bhargava, A., Shukla, S., and Ohri, D. (2006). Chenopodium quinoa: An Indian perspective. *Indus Crops Products* 23(1):73–87.

Borges, J. T. S., Ascheri, J. L. R., Ascheri, D. R., Nascimento, R. E., and Freitas, A. S. (2003). Propriedades de cozimento e caracterização físico-química de macarrão pré cozido à base de farinha integral de quinoa (Chenopodium quinoa Willd.) e de farinha de arroz (Oryza sativa, L.) polido por extrusão termoplástica. *Boletim do CEPPA* 21(2):303–322.

Borges, J. T. S., Bonomo, R. C., Paula, C. D., Oliveira, L. C., and Cesário, M. C. (2010). Physicochemical and nutritional characteristics and uses of Quinoa (Chenopodium quinoa Willd.). *Temas Agrários* 15(1):9–23.

Brady, K., Ho, C-T., Rosen, R. T., Sang, S., and Karwe, M. V. (2007). Effects of processing on the nutraceutical profile of quinoa. *Food Chem* 100(3):1209–1216.

Brinegar, C. and Goundan, S. (1993). Isolation and characterization of chenopodin, the 11S seed storage protein of quinoa (Chenopodium quinoa). *J Agric Food Chem* 41:182–185.

Brinegar, C., Sine, B., and Nwokocha, L. (1996). High-cysteine 2S seed storage proteins from Quinoa (Chenopodium quinoa). *J. Agric Food Chem* 44(7):1621–1623.

Chauhan, G. S., Eskin, N. A. M., and Tkachuk, R. (1992). Nutrients and antinutrients in quinoa seed. *Cereal Chem* 69:85–88.

Comai, S., Bertazzo, A., Bailoni, L., Zancato, M., Costa, C., and Allegri, G. (2007). The content of proteic and nonproteic (free and protein-bound) tryptophan in quinoa and cereal flours. *Food Chem* 100:1350–1355.

Coulter, L. and Lorenz, K. (1990). Quinoa-composition, nutritional value, food applications. *Lebensm Wiss u Technol* 23:203–207.

Cozolino, M. F. (2009). *Biodisponibilidade de Nutrientes*. 3ª Ed. Manole, Barueri, SP, Brazil, 1172 pp.

Cusack, D. (1984). Quinoa: Grain of the Incas. *Ecologist* 14:21–31.

Dini, I., Schettino, O., Simioli, T., and Dini, A. (2001). Studies on the constituents of *Chenopodium quinoa* seeds: Isolation and characterization of new triterpene saponins. *J Agric Food Chem* 49(2):741–746.

FAOSTAT. (2008). FAO Statistics, Food and Agriculture Organization of the United Nations. Rome, 2012. http://faostat.fao.org/site/567/DesktopDefault.aspx?PageID¼567#ancor.

Farro, P. C. A. (2008). Desenvolvimento de filmes biodegradáveis a partir de derivados do grão de quinoa (*Chenopodium quinoa* Willdenow) da variedade "Real." Thesis, Faculdade de Engenharia de Alimentos, Universidade Estadual de Campinas, Campinas, Brazil, 303 pp.

Francis, G., Kerem, Z., Makkar, H. P. S., and Becker, K. (2002). The biological action of saponins in animal systems: A review. *Br J Nutr* 88(6):587–605.

Gonzalez, J. A., Roldan, A., Gallardo, M., Escudero, T., and Prado, F. E. (1989). Quantitative determinations of chemical compounds with nutritional value from Inca crops: Chenopodium quinoa ('quinoa'). *Plant Foods Hum Nutr* 39(4):331–337.

Gorinstein, S., Lojek, A., Cîz, M., Pawelzik, E., Delgado-Licon, E., Medina, O. J., Moreno, M., Salas, I. A., and Goshev, I. (2008). Comparison of composition and antioxidant capacity of some cereals and pseudocereals. Int J Food Sci Technol 43(4):629–637.

Güçlü-Üstündag, Ö. and Mazza, G. (2007). Saponins: Properties, applications and processing. *Crit Rev Food Sci Nutr* 47(3):231–258.

Hirose, Y., Fujita, T., Ishii, T., and Ueno, N. (2010). Antioxidative properties and flavonoid composition of Chenopodium quinoa seeds cultivated in Japan. *Food Chem* 119(4):1300–1306.

Jacobsen, S. E., Jørgensen, I., and Stølen, O. (1994). Cultivation of quinoa (Chenopodium quinoa) under temperate climatic conditions in Denmark. *J Agric Sci* 122(1):47–52.

Jacobson, S. E., Mujica, A., and Jensen, C. (2003). The resistance of Quinoa (*Chenopodium quinoa Willd.*) to adverse abiotic factors. *Food Rev Int* 19(1–2):99–109. doi:10.1081/FRI-120018872

Jacobsen, S.-E. & Stolen, O. (1993). Quinoa – morphology, phenology and prospects for its production as a new crop in Europe. *Eur J Agron* 2:19–29.

Jancurová, M., Minarovičová, L., and Dandár, A. (2009). Quinoa – A review. *Czech J Food Sci* 27:71–79.

Karyotis, T., Iliadis, C., Noulas, C., and Mitsibonas, T. (2003). Preliminary research on seed production and nutrient content for certain quinoa varieties in a saline-sodic. *Soil J Agron Crop Sci* 189:402–408.

Khattab, R. Y. and Arntfield, S. D. (2009). Nutritional quality of legume seeds as affected by some physical treatments. 2. Antinutritional factors. *LWT Food Sci Technol* 42(6):1113–1118.

Konishi, Y., Hirano, S., Tsuboi, H., and Wada, M. (2004). Distribution of minerals in quinoa (Chenopodium quinoa Willd.) seeds. *Biosci Biotechnol Biochem* 68(1):231–234.

Koyro, H. W. and Eisa, S. (2007). Effect of salinity on composition, viability and germination of seeds of Chenopodium quinoa Willd. *Plant and Soil* 302(1):79–90.

Kozioł, M.J. (1990). Composicion quimica. In: *Quinua, hacia su cultivo commercial. Latinreco S.A., Casilla 17- 110–6053*. C. Wahli (Eds.). Quito, Equador, pp. 137–159.

Kozioł, M. J. (1992). Chemical composition and nutritional evaluation of quinoa (Chenopodium quinoa Willd.). *J Food Compos Anal* 5(1):35–68.

Kozioł, M. J. (1993). In: *Quinoa: A Potential New Oil Crop. New Crops*. J. Janick and J. E. Simon (Eds.). Wiley, New York, pp. 328–336.

Kuljanabhagavad, T., Thongphasuk, P., Chamulitrat, W., and Wink, M. (2008). Triterpene saponins from Chenopodium quinoa Willd. *Phytochemistry* 69:1919–1926.

Lorenz, K. (1990). Quinoa (*Chenopodium quinoa*) starch – Physico-chemical properties and functional characteristics. *Starch* 42(3):81–86.

Lopes, C. O., Dessimoni, G. V., Da Silva, M. C., Vieira, G., and Pinto, N. A. V. D. (2009). Aproveitamento, composição nutricional e antinutricional da farinha de quinoa (Chenoipodium quinoa). Alimentos e Nutrição 20(4):669–675.

Lorenz, K., Coulter, L., and Johnson, D. (1995). Functional and sensory characteristics of quinoa in foods. *Dev Food Sci* 37:1031–1041.

Mahan, L. K. and Escott-Stump, S. (2010). *Krause—Alimentos, Nutrição e Dietoterapia*. 12th ed. Elsevier, Rio de Janeiro, 1351 pp.

Marticorena, C. and Quezada, M. (1985). *Gayana Botánica* 42, 1–2. Universitaria Ed. Concepción, pp. 28 and 146.

Masson, L. and Mella, M. A. (1985). Materials grassas de consume habitual y Potential en Chile. (Ed. Universitaria), pp. 23. Santiago.{Minerals in quinoa (Chenopodium quinoa Willd.) seeds.

Mastebroek, H. D., Limburg, H., Gilles, T., and Marvin, H. J. P. (2000). Occurrence of sapogenins in leaves and seeds of quinoa (*Chenopodium quinoa* Willd). *J Food Sci Agri* 80(1):152–156.

Meyer, B., Heinstein, P., Burnouf-Radosevich, M., Delfel, N., and McLaughlin, J. (1990). Bioactivity-directed isolation and characterization of quinoside a: One of the toxic/bitter principles of quinoa seeds (*Chenopodium quinoa* Willd.). *J Agric Food Chem* 38:205–208.

Miranda, M., Vega-Gálvez, A., Quispe-Fuentes, I., Rodríguez, M. J., Maureira, H., and Martínez, E. A. (2012). Nutritional aspects of six quinoa (Chenopodium quinoa Willd.) ecotypes from three geographical areas of Chile. *Chilean J Agri Res* 72:175–181.

Mujica, A., Chura, E., Ruiz, E., Rossel, J., and Pocco, M. (2010). Mecanismos de resitencia a sales y seleccion de variedades de quinua (Chenopodium quinoa Willd.) resistates a salinidad. In: Anales XII Congraso Nacional de las Ciencias del Suelo y V Congresso Internacional de las Ciencias del Suelo, Arequipa, Peru, 11–15 October, pp. 187–189.

Mujica, A., Jacobsen, S. E., Ezquierdo, J., and Marathee, J. P. (2001). *Resultados de la Prueba Americana y Europes de la Quinua*. FAO, UNA-Puno, CIP, Santiago, p. 51.

Nara, S. and Komiya, T. (1983). Studies on the relationship between water-saturated state and crystallinity by the diffraction method for moistened potato starch. *Starch* 35:407–410.

Ng, S., Anderson, A., Coker, J., and Ondrus, M. (2007). Characterization of lipid oxidation products in quinoa (*Chenopodium quinoa*). *Food Chem* 101(1):185–192.

Nowak, V., Du, J., and Charrondière, U. R. (2015). Assessment of the nutritional composition of quinoa (Chenopodium quinoa Wild). *Food Chem* 193:47–54.

Nsimba, R. Y., Kikuzaki, H., and Konishi, Y. (2008). Antioxidant activity of various extracts and fractions of Chenopodium quinoa and Amaranthus spp. seeds. Food Chem 106(2):760–766.

Ogungbenle, H. N. (2003). Nutritional evaluation and functional properties of quinoa (Chenopodium quinoa) flour. *Int J Food Sci Nutr* 54(2):153–158.

Oliveira, A. C., Reis, S. M. P. M., Carvalho, E. M., Pimenta, F. M. V., Rios, K. R., Paiva, K. C., Sousa, L. M., Almeida, M., and Arruda, S. F. (2003). Adições crescentes de ácido fitico à dieta não interferiram na digestibilidade da caseína e no ganho de peso em ratos. *Revista de Nutrição* 16(2):211–217.

Oshodi, A. A., Ogungbenle, H. N., and Oladimeji, M. O. (1999). Chemical composition, nutritionally valuable minerals and functional properties of benniseed (Sesamum radiatum), pearl millet (Pennisetum typhoides) and quinoa (Chenopodium quinoa) flours. *Int J Food Sci Nutr* 50(5):325–331.

Park, J. K. et al. (2007). The miRNA pathway intrinsically controls self-renewal of Drosophila germline stem cells. *Curr Biol* 17(6):533–538.

Park, S. H. and Naofumi, M. (2004). Changes of bound lipids and composition of fatty acids in germination of quinoa seeds. *Food Sci Technol* 10(3):303–306.

Praznik, W., Mundigler, N., Kogler, A., Pelzl, B., and Huber, A. (1999). Molecular background of technological properties of selected starches. *Starch* 51:197–211.

Qian, J. Y. and Kuhn, M. (1999). Characterization of Amaranthus cruentus and Chenopodium quinoa starch. *Starch* 51:116–120.

Repo-Carrasco, R., Espinoza, C., and Jacobsen, S. (2003). Nutritional value and use of the Andean crops quinoa (Chenopodium quinoa) and kan˜iwa (Chenopodium pallidicaule). *Food Rev Int* 19:179–189.

Ruales, J., Grijalva, Y., Jaramillo, P. L., and Nair, B. M. (2002). The nutritional quality of an infant food from quinoa and its effect on the plasma level of insulin-like growth factor-I (IGF-I) in undernourished children. *Int J Food Sci Nutr* 53(2):143–154.

Ruales, J. and Nair, B. M. (1992). Nutritional quality of the protein in quinoa (Chenopodium quinoa Willd) seeds. *Plant Foods Hum Nutr* 42:1–12.

Ruales, J. and Nair, B. M. (1993). Content of fat, vitamins and minerals in quinoa (Chenopodium quinoa Willd.) seeds. *Food Chem* 48:131–136.

Ruales, J. and Nair, B. M. (1993b). Saponins, phytic acid, tannis and protease inhibitors in quinoa (Chenopodium quinoa Willd) seeds. Food Chem 48(2):137–143.

Ruales, J. and Nair, B. M. (1994). Properties of starch and dietary fiber in raw and processed quinoa (Chenopodium quinoa, Willd.) seeds. *Plant Foods Human Nutr* 45:223–246.

Ruiz, K. B., Biondi, S., Oses, R., Acuña-Rodríguez, I. S., Antognoni, F., Martinez-Mosqueira, E. A., et al. (2014). Quinoa biodiversity and sustainability for food security under climate change: A review. *Agron Sustain Dev* 34:349–359.

von Rütte, S., and Usos. (1990). Chap. IX. In: *Quinua hacia su Cultivo Comercial*. C. Wahli (Ed.). Quito, Latinreco, SA, pp. 161–168.

Ryan, E., Galvin, K., O'Connor, T. P., and Maguire, A. R. (2007). Phytosterol, squalene, tocopherol content and fatty acid profile of selected seeds, grains, and legumes. *Plant Foods Hum Nutr* 62(3):85–91.

Santos, M. A. T. (2006). Efeito do cozimento sobre alguns fatores antinutricionais em folhas de brocou, couve-flor e couve. *Ciência e Agrotecnologia* 30(2):294–301.

Seeman, P., Cheng, D., and Iles, G. (1973). Structure of membrane holes in osmotic and saponin hemolysis. *J Cell Biol* 56:519–527.

Simopoulos, A. (1991). Omega-3 fatty acids in health and disease and in growth and development. *Am J Clin Nutr* 54:438–463.

Singer, N. S., Tang, P., Chang, H., and Dunn, J. M. (1990). Carbohydrate cream substitute. U.S. Patent 4911946 A.

Souza, L. A. C., Spehar, C. R., and Santos, R. L. B. (2004). Análise de imagem para determinação do teor de saponina em quinoa. *Pesquisa Agropecuária Brasileira* 39(4):397–401.

Sparg, S., Light, M., and van Staden, J. (2004). Biological activities and distribution of plant saponins. *J Ethnopharmacol* 94(2–3):219–243.

Spehar, C. R. (2006). Adaptação da Quinoa (Chenopodium quinoa Willd.) para incrementar a diversidade agrícola e alimentar no Brasil. *Cadernos de Ciência & Tecnologia* 23(1):41–62.

Spehar, C. R. (2007). *Quinoa: alternativa para a diversificação agrícola e alimentar*. Ed. Técnico. Embrapa Cerrados, Planaltina, DF, p. 103.

Spehar, C. R. and Santos, R. L. B. (2002). Quinoa 'BRS Piabiru': alternativa para diversificar os sistemas de produção de grãos. *Pesquisa Agropecuária Brasileira* 37(6):889–893.

Stevens, J. M. (1994). Orach-Atriplex hortensis L. Fact sheet HS-637, Horticultural Sciences Department, Florida Cooperative Extension Service, Inst. Food and Agricultural Sciences. University of Florida: Gainesville.

Stuardo, M. and San Martin, R. (2008). Antifungal properties of quinoa (*Chenopodium quinoa* Willd.) alkali treated previous termsaponinsnext term against Botrytis cinerea. *Ind Crops Prod* 27(3):296–302.

Tang, Y., Li, X., Chen, P. X., Zhang, B., Hernandez, M., et al. (2014). Lipids, tocopherols, and carotenoids in leaves of amaranth and quinoa cultivars and a new approach to overall evaluation of nutritional quality traits. *J Agric Food Chem* 62:12610–12619.

Tang, Y., Li, X., Chen, P. X., Zhang, B., Hernandez, M., et al. (2015a). Characterisation of fatty acid, carotenoid, tocopherol/tocotrienol compositions and antioxidant activities in seeds of three Chenopodium quinoa Willd. genotypes. *Food Chem* 174:502–508.

Tang, Y., Li, X., Zhang, B., Chen, P. X., Liu, R., et al. (2015b). Characterisation of phenolics, betanins and antioxidant activities in seeds of three Chenopodium quinoa Willd. genotypes. *Food Chem* 166:380–388.

Tang, Y., Lu, A., Aronow, B. J., Wagner, K. R., Sharp, F. R. (2002). Genomic responses of the brain to ischemic stroke, intracerebral haemorrhage, kainate seizures, hypoglycemia, and hypoxia. Eur J Neurosci 15:1937–1952.

Tapia, M. E. (1979). Historia y Distribucion geographica. Quinua y Kaniwa. Cultivos Andinos. In: *Serie Libros y Materiales Educativos*, Vol. 5. M. E. Tapia (Ed.). Instituto Interamericano de Ciencias Agricolas, Bogota, Colombia, pp. 11–15.

Tapia, M. (1982). *The environment, crops and agricultural systems in the Andes and Southern Peru*. IICA.

Tari, T. A., Annapure, U. S., Singhal, R. S., and Kulkarni, P. R. (2003). Starch-based spherical aggregates: screening of small granule sized starches for entrapment of a model flavouring compound, vanillin. *Carbohydr Polym* 53:45–51.

Tari, T. A. and Singhal, R. S. (2002). Starch-based spherical aggregates: Stability of a model flavouring compound, vanillin entrapped therein. *Carbohydr Polym* 50:417–421.

Tavakkoli-Kakhki, M., Motavasselian, M., Mosaddegh, M., Mahdi Esfahani, M., Kamalinejad, M., Nematy, M., and Eslami, S. (2014). Omega-3 and omega-6 content of medicinal foods for depressed patients: Implications from the Iranian Traditional Medicine. *Avicenna J Phytomed* 4(4):225–230.

United States Department of Agriculture (USDA) – Agricultural Research Service. (2011). National Nutrient Database for Standard Reference, Release 27. Nutrient Data Laboratory. Available from: http://www.nal.usda.gov/fnic/foodcomp/search. Accessed 15 August 2014.

USDA U.S. Department of Agriculture, Agricultural Research Service. (2005). USDA National Nutrient Database for Standard Reference, Release 18. Nutrient Data Laboratory Home Page, http://www.ars.usda.gov/nutrientdata.

USDA U.S. Department of Agriculture, Agricultural Research Service. (2018). USDA National Nutrient Database for Standard Reference, Release 18. Nutrient Data Laboratory Home Page, http://www.ars.usda.gov/nutrientdata/flav.

Vega-Galvez, A., Miranda, M., Vergara, J., Uribe, E., Puente, L., and Martinez, E. A. (2010). Nutrition facts and functional potential of quinoa (*Chenopodium quinoa* Willd.), an ancient Andean grain: A review. *J Sci Food Agri* 90(15):2541–2547.

Wilson, H. D. (1980). Artificial hybridization among species of Chenopodium sect. Chenopodium. *Syst Bot* 5:253–263.

Wilson, H. D. (1981). Genetic variation among South American populations of tetraploid Chenopodium sect. Chenopodium subsect. Cellulata. *Syst Bot* 6(4). American Society of Plant Taxonomists. https://doi.org/10.2307/2418450

Wilson, H. D. (1988a). Allozyme variation and morphological relationships of Chenopodium hircinum Schrader (s. lat.). *Syst Bot* 13:215–228. https://doi.org/10.2307/2419100

Wilson, H. D. (1988b). Quinua biosystematics I. Domestic populations. *Econ Bot* 42:461–477.

Wilson, H. D. (1990). Quinua and relatives (Chenopodium sect. Chenopodium subsect. Cellulata. *Econ Bot* 44:92–110.

Wilson, C., Read, J. J., and Abo, K. E. (2002). Effect of mixed-salt salinity on growth and ion relations of a quinoa and a wheat variety. *J Plant Nutr* 25(12):2689–2704.

Winkel, T., Flores, R. Á., Bertero, D., Cruz, P., del Castillo, C., Joffre, R., Parada, S. P., and Tonacca, L. S. (2014). Calling for a reappraisal of the impact of quinoa expansion on agricultural sustainability in the Andean highlands. *Idesia* 32:95–100.

Woldemichael, G. M. and Wink, M. (2001). Identification and biological activities of triterpenoid saponins from Chenopodium quinoa. *J Agric Food Chem* 49(5):2327–2332.

Wood, S. G., Lawson, L. D., Fairbanks, D. J., Robinson, L. R., and Anderson, W. R. (1993). Seed lipid content and fatty acid composition of three quinoa cultivars. *J Food Comp Anal* 6:41–44.

Wright, K. H., Huber, K. C., Fairbanks, D. J., and Huber, C. S. (2002a). Isolation and characterization of Atriplex hortensis and sweet Chenopodium quinoa starches. *Cereal Chem* 79(5):715–719.

Wright, K. H., Pike, O. A., Fairbanks, D. J., and Huber, C. S. (2002b). Composition of atriplex hortensis, sweet and bitter *Chenopodium quinoa* seeds. *J Food Sci* 67(4):1383–1385.

Youdim, K., Martin, A., and Joseph, J. (2000). Essential fatty acids and the brain: Possible health implications. *Int J Dev Neurosci* 18(4–5):383–399.

Zhu, N., Sheng, S., Li, D., Lavoie, E. J., Karwe, M. V., Rosen, R. T., and Ho, C-T. (2001). Antioxidative flavonoid glycosides from quinoa seeds (Chenopodium Quinoa). *J Food Lipids* 8(1):37–44.

Zhu, N., Sheng, S., Sang, S., Jhoo, J.-W., Bai, N., Karwe, M. V., Rosen, R. T., and Ho, C.-T. (2002). Triterpene Saponins from Debittered Quinoa (Chenopodium quinoa) Seeds. J Agric Food Chem 50(4):865–867.

3 Physical, Chemical, and Functional Properties of Chia

To ensure an adequate supply of nutrients to complement the standard diet, consumption of super seeds such as *Salvia hispanica* L., commonly known as chia seeds, is rapidly increasing. Chia seeds are known as an excellent source of fat (20%–35%), particularly polyunsaturated fatty acids such as α-linolenic (58%–60%) and linoleic (18%–20%) acids. Moreover, high protein levels (16%–25%), mainly prolamins, and dietary fiber contents (23%–40%) have been reported. Vitamins, mostly B complex, and minerals including calcium, magnesium, phosphorus, and potassium have also been found in significant amounts.

Additionally, due to the absence of gluten, chia seeds are appropriate for celiac patients. Regarding other bioactive compounds, chia seeds are a good source of antioxidants, such as chlorogenic and caffeic acids, quercetin, and kaempferol. Due to their described composition, chia seeds have been related to different medicinal effects, particularly anti-inflammatory and antidiabetic activities, and positive effects on cardiovascular disease and hypertension. This chapter systematically reviews the components of chia seeds to update their morphology, chemical composition, and possibly human health benefits.

Chia seeds are currently consumed due to their potential health benefits. The isoflavones present in chia seeds (with average contents of daidzin 0.0066, glycitin 0.0014, genistin 0.0034, glycitein 0.0005, and genistein 0.0051 mg/g of seed) may be used as a new source for the treatment of several disorders. These substances can be recognized as anticarcinogenic, with potential therapeutic applications in the prevention of cardiovascular disease. More specifically, phytoestrogens are considered to exhibit estrogenic activity. These are usually used to treat menopause symptoms, postmenopause, osteoporosis, and other estrogen-related disorders. The high fiber content in chia may convey health benefits because fiber can help increase stool volume and prevent diseases such as diverticulosis and cancer. Fiber can also help slow the digestion process and the release of glucose, providing antidiabetic effects. Moreover, it improves the peristaltic movements of the intestines and decreases plasma cholesterol. In 2007, Espada et al. subjected Wistar rats to twice-daily administration of 25 g of chia seed or powder mixed in 0.25 L of water; they registered significant tumor weight decreases in the chia oil group compared to the control group (maintained on a commercial diet). This behavior was not observed in the safflower (*Carthamus tinctorius* L.) oil group. Furthermore, the chia oil diet encouraged apoptosis and discouraged mitosis. Its membranes had higher contents of EPA, although those from the safflower oil group had higher contents of ALA

DOI: 10.1201/9781003080770-3

than the control and chia groups. EPA appears to have a direct apoptotic effect, stimulating caspase activity and, consequently, programmed cell death; thus, it has antitumor potential. Ayerza and Coates evaluated the immune stimulant activity of chia seeds; they reported numerous advantages over other Ω-3 PUFA products in relieving various conditions, such as diarrhea, allergies, weight loss, and digestive problems. Chia had similar effects to fish oil on parameters such as food intake, body weight, thymus weight, thymocyte number, and immunoglobin E levels. The hydrolysis of chia protein creates low molecular weight peptides with antioxidant activities and inhibitory potential of ACE. The antioxidant potentials of different chia olein fractions were evaluated; the control was 100% milk fat, and the chia olein fractions corresponded to 5%, 10%, 15%, and 20% chia olein completed with milk fat. The values obtained for the control group and the four different fractions were 5.62%, 17.42%, 36.83%, 51.18%, and 74.94%, respectively, evidencing improvements in 2,2-diphenyl-1-picrylhydrazyl free radical scavenging activity. It was suggested that chia seeds could act as an electron donor and scavenger for free radicals as chia protein isolates showed inhibitory effects on angiotensin-converting enzymes that were also far more potent than in *Phaseolus lunatus* L. and *Phaseolus vulgaris* L. (Fabaceae). Moreover, peptides fractioned from prolamins and globulin could participate effectively in the *in vitro* chelation of ferrous ion (Fe^{2+}) in a gastrointestinal tract simulation. Chia also evidenced antiradical activity against 2,2′-azinobis (3-ethylbenzothiazoline 6-sulfonic acid) and 2,2-diphenyl-1-picrylhydrazyl well as angiotensin-converting enzyme activity. In obese rats treated with chia seed and its oils; insulin and glucose tolerance improvements, visceral adiposity, hepatic steatosis, cardiac and hepatic fibrosis, and inflammation were verified. Chia seed inhibits the activity of SCD, which is responsible for the conversion of elaidic acid to its conjugate, linolenic acid. The study proposes that linoleic acid is oxidized and carried to the mitochondria, downregulating the n-6/n-3 ratio. The inhibition of SCD prevents obesity, cellular lipid accumulation, and insulin resistance due to a decrease in the expression of the SCD promoter. This happens because SCD produces plasma palmitoleate, which is associated with human hypertriglyceridemia and abdominal adiposity. However, body-weight gain, abdominal fat growth, and food intake did not decrease in this study. Only the 6-week treatment decreased the levels of heat shock proteins (HSPs) 60 and 70, although no changes in the levels of HSPs 25 and 90 were observed. Although either of these treatments did not alter catalase, lipase, and dihydrofolate reductase levels, treatment with chia oil could change glutathione peroxidase levels. The SOD content increased, but not to normal control levels. In 2015, Marinelli et al. supported the metabolic pathway proposed by Poudyal et al. (2012). In Marinelli's work, also with obese rats, it was indicated that concerning the high fructose group (administered 4% soybean oil, 31% lard, and 20% fructose), chia seeds did not decrease fat accumulation or body weight gain despite having positive effects on glucose.

The beneficial effects of high contents of bioactive compounds in food products depend on their intake and composition (especially polyphenol compounds, which are directly related to antioxidant properties) and alteration of the contents during digestion. A study evaluated the indices of recovery and bioaccessibility of phenols and flavonoids and their corresponding antioxidant capacity during

TABLE 3.1
Properties of Chia Seeds

Functional Component	Nutritional Value	Health/Medical Value	Technological Functionality
Whole chia seed	Gluten-free, polyunsaturated fatty acids, proteins, dietary fiber, vitamins, antioxidants and minerals. No evidence of adverse effects and no indication of allergenicity	Long-therm supplementation attenuates cardiovascular risk in people with diabetes type 2. Reduction of postprandial glycemia and prolongation of satiety.	Production of bread, cookies, cereal bars, yogurt and others.
Proteins	High quality of protein due to the content of the nine essential aminoacids: leucine, isoleucine, lysine, methionine, phenylalanine, threonine, tryptophan, valine and histidine.	Potential source of bioactive peptides. Usefulness for specific vital purposes: growth, replacement of metabolic losses and damage tissue, reproduction, lactation and general well-being.	Potential production of health-enhancing ingredients to improve functional foods.
Fatty acids	Rich in alpha-linolenic fatty acid	Capable of preventing the the onset of dyslipidemia in rats. It helps to reduce the cholesterol. Regulation of blood pressure and plasma triglyceride concentration. The presence of n-3 fatty acids and antioxidants in chia seeds could promote a reduction in the inflammatory response.	Chia essential oil encapsulation for uses as nutraceutical Production of omega-enriched eggs
Mucilage	Production of fiber-enriched foods. Increase postmeal satiety.	It helps to reduce the digestion time of carbohydrates.	Ability to achieve water control and modulate texture in a vast range of food products. Mucilage can replace as much as 25% of oil or eggs in cake and can produce edible films in combination with whey protein concentrate. Can also act such as thickener, foaming and emulsifying agent

(*Continued*)

TABLE 3.1 (*Continued*)
Properties of Chia Seeds

Functional Component	Nutritional Value	Health/Medical Value	Technological Functionality
Others	Good proportions of tocopherol and sterols antioxidants, vitamins and minerals.		Important source of antioxidants with commercial applications

Source: USDA National Nutrient Database for Standard Reference, Release 24 (2011)

in vitro gastrointestinal digestion of nondefatted and defatted chia seeds. Simulations of the various digestion phases, namely oral, gastric and intestinal, were required to achieve the proposed aim. To this end, extractions of undigested and digested samples were performed, and the total phenolic compounds (TPCs), total flavonoid content (TFC), and antioxidant capacity were determined. Finally, the recovery (RI) and bioaccessibility (BI) indices were calculated. Concerning the results, there were no significant differences in the RI between the nondefatted and defatted samples after the three mimicked digestion phases. However, the oral phase negatively affects phenol recovery because the RI was lower than the test matrix used as a reference in both samples. Despite this, the RI had the highest recovery results; this indicates a release of compounds from the matrix in the gastric phase, probably due to gastric acidic and alkaline hydrolysis. The bioaccessibility of phenolic acids was higher than that of flavonoids in the case of nondefatted chia, even though similar values were obtained for defatted chia. For the TFC, no statistical differences were observed, although the defatted chia had a lower recovery after the intestinal stage than the nondefatted sample. There was also a decrease in the RI after the oral phase with the reference. The TFC was affected by the gastrointestinal digestion process because, after digestion, the recovery increased for nondefatted chia similarly to the reference matrix but not for the defatted sample, which had a similar recovery to the gastric phase; this may be related to the low stability and interaction of flavonoids with the food matrix compounds. The different responses of defatted and nondefatted samples to gastrointestinal digestion may result from the fat content, where higher fat contents retain flavonoids and affect the digestion process of the samples. The BI for phenolic acids was higher than that of flavonoids for nondefatted chia, while defatted chia showed similar values. In general, the concentration of polyphenolic compounds increased during digestion; however, only low medium and low percentages of phenols and flavonoids, respectively, were available for absorption in the intestinal tract. Additionally, the presence of high levels of fat appears to impact the bioaccessibility of flavonoids negatively. The divergence of the correlation results obtained between the TPC, TFC, and antioxidant capacity should also be noted. Low bioaccessibility values were obtained for both phenols and flavonoids; however, their potential antioxidant capacity supports using nondefatted and defatted chia seeds as food ingredients. Further research is required to describe the stabilities of chia bioactive compounds and improve their bioaccessibility. Regarding the functionality of chia protein hydrolysates, they were obtained with the Alcalase-Flavourzyme sequential enzymatic system and exhibited ACE inhibitory activity, suggesting that these peptides are responsible for ACE inhibition; however, it depends upon the hydrolysis time and the degree of hydrolysis (DH). The fact that these hydrolysates are resistant to gastrointestinal proteases allows their incorporation into food systems. The hydrolysates also underwent single-electron transfer reactions in the ABTS+ reduction assay, in which they most likely acted as electron donors and free radical sinks, therefore providing antioxidant protection. However, this should be confirmed for each peptide in different oxidant systems and under *in vitro* and *in vivo* conditions. No relationship between antioxidant activity and the hydrolysates with the highest ACE inhibitory activity was found. This implies that peptide antioxidant activity depends on the specific proteases that produce the peptides, the obtained DH, the molecular weights, compositions, amino acid sequences of the peptides, and the combined effects of free radical location capacity, metal ion chelation, and electron donation. Overall, the DH is the major factor affecting their potential biological activity levels in chia protein hydrolysates. A higher DH value results in higher ACE inhibitory activity; this was not observed for the antioxidant activity, which was lowered. These peptides with ACE inhibitory and antioxidant activities should be incorporated as ingredients in functional foods. Regarding *S. hispanica* safety, the UK Committee for Novel Foods and Processes reported potential protein allergenicity by specific IgE binding and immunoblotting. It has been proposed that chia-containing products should carry advisories for consumers with food sensitivities, particularly to sesame and mustard seeds, because cross-reactivity may occur. However, the toxicological safety of *S. hispanica* was accessed and considered satisfactory in a 4-week study involving 100 healthy subjects divided into four groups and given either 4 g sunflower seeds (control) or 2.5 g, 5 g, or 10 g of chia seeds per day. No significant adverse effects have been reported. Despite this, chia seed may lower blood pressure (antihypertensive effect); therefore, its supplementation should be used carefully in patients with hypotension or taking blood pressure medication and cases with type II diabetes.

Due to inclusion of chia seed oil in dietary supplements, in December 2017, it was included in the United States Pharmacopeia; since then, it has been regarded as safe. Chia seed oil is the oil extracted from chia seeds by cold pressing, excluding the extraction methods that include solvent use or external heat. A public quality standard was also established to ensure quality product delivery by manufacturers, and the addition of tocopherols was recommended for oil preservation. The chemical characteristics of chia seed oil were analyzed, and the following results were reported: iodine value 207, saponification index 193.3, and tocopherol content 480 mg/kg. The copper and iron contents were 0.1 and 0.3 ppm, respectively. The peroxide and anisidine values were 1.0 and 0.3 meq O2 per kg, respectively. The induction period in a Rancimat was 2.3 h, and the oil yield was 35.6–38.6. Different techniques for seed oil extraction, namely seed compression with cold pressing at 4°C or Komet screw pressing at 25°C–30°C with electrical resistance heating (preserves antioxidant contents better than solvent extraction only recovers part of the oil). It can also be done with solvents, using the Soxhlet method with *n*-hexane, which favors water holding, organic molecule absorption and capacity, and emulsifying stability, but loses antioxidants.

Furthermore, supercritical fluids, such as carbon dioxide at a pressure of 408 bar and temperature of 80°C (better purity and higher ALA/LA contents were obtained in the final products). Chia coproduct remaining after the oil extraction process by cold-pressing was analyzed, and higher levels of proteins and total dietary fiber (TDF) content than in chia seeds were found. Its composition suggests its suitability as an ingredient for food formulations because it still contains high biological value proteins and fiber but has a lower energy value.

Furthermore, the higher level of polyphenolic compounds than in chia seeds demonstrates its higher antioxidant activity. In terms of its functional properties, the chia coproduct is similar to chia seeds. Apart from decreases in the water holding capacity and gelling capacity, parameters are essential in applications such as producing gelled products cooked meat foods. After the extraction of chia seed oil, significant portions of dietary fiber (~33.9 g per 100 g) and protein (~17 g per 100 g) remain. The low oxidative stability of chia seed oil represents a technological disadvantage. However, when exposed to environmental factors (light and oxygen), it contains natural antioxidant compounds, compromising its chemical quality and decreasing its shelf life. Adding additional antioxidants can address the issue. A study evaluated storage condition effects at room temperature for 300 days under fluorescent light (800 Lux) or in the dark. Under the protective effects of combined ascorbyl palmitate and tocopherol (50:50, natural antioxidants) were more effective than tertiary-butyl hydroquinone (synthetic antioxidant), maintaining acceptable quality for at least 300 days. Chia seeds are an essential source of fat (namely polyunsaturated fatty acids, such as α-linolenic and linoleic acids), protein, especially prolamins, carbohydrates, insoluble fiber, vitamins (mainly from B complex), minerals (such as calcium, phosphorus, or potassium), and antioxidants (chlorogenic and caffeic acids, quercetin, or kaempferol). Thus, chia seeds and their by-products (such as oil and flour) are increasingly incorporated into different food products.

Chia seeds have a significant role as a functional food and nutritional supplement (Coelho et al., 2018). The composition and the concentration of their bioactive compounds depend on several factors such as climatic conditions, geographical origin, and extraction methods (Ayerza and Coates, 2005, 2009, 2011; Capitani et al., 2012; Ixtaina et al., 2011). Seeds are composed of TDF from 47.3% to 59.9% (Weber et al., 1991) and contain up to 38%–40% of oil with high content of unsaturated fatty acids. Moreover, they are also a good source of proteins (18.8%–27.1%), dietary fiber, vitamins, minerals, and antioxidants (Bushway et al., 1981). Compared to other grains, chia seeds do not contain toxic compounds and gluten, making seeds a safe ingredient for gluten-free diets (Menga et al., 2017).

Caffeic acid from chia seed extract plays an important role in contributing to both chemical and biological properties. Caffeic acid is also classified as hydroxycinnamic acid, and it can be bound to quinic acid in different positions to give rise to a class of metabolites called caffeoylquinic acids. Among all of these, chlorogenic acid is the most common abundant in the polar extract of chia seeds (Martínez-Cruz and Paredes-López, 2014). Various researchers have found a concentration of caffeic acid (0.0276 mg/g) higher than that reported for mango (0.0076 mg/g), papaya

TABLE 3.2
Mineral Content (per 100 g)

Macroelements

Nutrient	Mg
Calcium	631
Potassium	407
Magnesium	335
Phosphorus	860
Microelements	**(μg)**
Selenium	55.2
Copper	0.924
Iron	7.72
Manganese	2.723
Molybdenum	0.2
Sodium	16
Zinc	4.58

Source: USDA National Nutrient Database for Standard Reference, Release 24 (2011)

TABLE 3.3
Vitamin Content (per 100 g)

Vitamins	Quantity (Units)
Vitamin C (total ascorbic acid)	1.6 mg
Thiamine	0.62 mg
Riboflavin	0.17 mg
Niacin	8.83 mg
Folate	49 μg
Vitamin A	54 IU
Vitamin E (alpha-tocopherol)	0.5 mg

Source: USDA National Nutrient Database for Standard Reference, Release 24 (2011),
IU: International unit

(0.0170 mg/g), and blueberry (0.0217mg/g), but found much lower than for peach (0.0371 mg/g) (Balasundram et al., 2006). Ayerza (2013), after HPLC analysis, also reported that chlorogenic acid is the most abundant phenol (0.224 mg/g) followed by caffeic acid (0.146 mg/g). Martínez-Cruz and Paredes-López, in the year 2014, reported that rosmarinic acid is the major phenolic compound of chia seeds (0.9271 mg/g). When the detailed analysis was done, it was found that trimers and tetramers of caffeic acid building block, including salvianolic acid A–K and lithospermic acid, may also be extracted from other Salvia species such as *S. miltiorrhiza*, *S. officinalis*,

S. cavaleriei, *S. flava*, *S. chinensis* as reported by Ai et al., in the year 1994; and later confirmed by Lu and Foo in the year 2001.

Flavonoids are the ubiquitous compounds present in plants. These belong to a polyphenolic subclass with a 15 carbon skeleton consisting of mainly two benzene rings linked via a heterocyclic pyrene ring (C). They are the compounds responsible for taste, color, and prevention of fat oxidation in food (Yao et al., 2004). Flavonoids possess many biochemical activities such as antioxidant, hepatoprotective, antibacterial, anti-inflammatory, anticancer, and antiviral (Cushnie and Lamb, 2005; Li et al., 2000; Zandi et al., 2011; Zhu et al., 2012).

Since ancient times, oil is extracted from chia seeds, which has been used in traditional medicine to get protection from eye infections and the treatment of stomach disorders (Lu and Foo, 2002; Reyes-Caudillo et al., 2008). Researchers demonstrated that oil extracted from chia seeds also contains phenolic compounds such as carotenoids, tocopherols, and phytosterols with antioxidant activity that play a crucial role in lipid oxidation (Matthaus, 2002; Ixtaina et al., 2011). Oil extracted from Italian varieties of chia seeds was not significantly different from that cultivated in Peru and Australia. However, the oil extracted from chia seeds grown in Italy was richer in chlorophyll, carotenoids, and α-linolenic acid but showed a higher free acidity and peroxides. As mentioned previously by various researchers, the chemical composition and oil yield can be affected by many factors such as extraction techniques and geographical area. In the year 2011, Ixtaina et al. used two extraction techniques to obtain oil from chia seeds purchased from Argentina and Guatemala. In both the varieties of seeds, the oil yield was much lower in pressing than in solvent extraction (20.3% and 24.8% compared to 26.70% and 33.6%, respectively). Dabrowski et al. (2016) also studied the effects of various extraction methods on the constituents and composition of chia seed oil. It was found that the recovery of oil was less by pressing method than done by extraction methods. Studies were also conducted to see the effect of different environments of South America on the protein content and oil contents, fatty acid composition, and peroxide index of chia seeds from Argentina (Ayerza and Coates, 2004; Ayerza, 2013). The researchers stated in the results that the chemical composition of the seeds is widely affected by the location and environmental factors, including temperature, light, and soil type.

Olivos-Lugo et al., in the year 2010, studied the nutritional, thermal, and functional by advanced techniques and provided data for properties like gelling, foaming water-holding capacity, and oil-holding capacity, amino-acid profile, and chemical score along with *in vitro* digestibility tests. They found that the protein fractions are composed of albumins (38 g/kg protein), globulins (71 g/kg protein), prolamins (537 g/kg protein), and also glutelins (229 g/kg protein). Ayerza and Coates (2011) studied the effect of altitude on the protein quality of seeds and found a gradual decrease of protein content as the altitude of the seed grown location increased. The denaturation temperatures of crude albumins, prolamins, globulins, and glutelins were 104°C, 86.5°C, 106°C, and 92°C. This indicates good thermal stability for albumins and globulins.

Chia seeds are a potential ingredient in the food industry because of their dietary fiber content. Nowadays, the definition is broader, including the plant components and all the carbohydrate polymers (Codex Alimentarius Commission, 2009). Dietary fiber is a compound that includes oligosaccharides and polysaccharides such as celluloses and hemicellulose. These may be associated with other components such as lignin, pectins, gums, and mucilage. The TDF has potential effects on the swelling property after water absorption. This is because carbohydrates with free polar groups that interact with hydrophilic links within the matrix lead to gel formation and consequent increase of peristalsis. Many published reports confirm the many health benefits are associated with the intake of TDF. The fiber provides a prebiotic effect to the diet, and it is effective for coronary heart disease, stroke, diabetes, hypertension, obesity, and many gastrointestinal disorders (Lairon et al., 2005; Montonen et al., 2003; Petruzziello et al., 2006; Whelton et al., 2005). Chia seeds are a good source of TDF, composed of soluble dietary fiber (SDF) and insoluble dietary fiber (IDF). Notably, the SDF is partially expelled from the seed as a mucilaginous gel when it comes in contact with water and is fermented in the colon (Anderson et al., 2009). The highest amount of the insoluble fiber-rich fraction (FRF) was also detected in *S. hispanica* seeds from Mexico by Vazquez-Ovando et al. (2009). Mainly they evaluated the FRF obtained by dry processing of defatted flour of chia seeds and reported 29.66 g/100 g of crude fiber content, 57.47 g/100 g of TDF content, of which 54.41 g/100 g was IDF, and 3.02 g/100 g was SDF. Compared to other reports, these values clearly show that dry fractionation with 100 mesh effectively concentrated TDF content. A part of the fiber in chia is located in the outer cells of the fruit. It is partly extruded from the fruit surface upon hydration in the form of a clear mucilaginous capsule that adheres firmly to the fruit itself.

The risks of chronic diseases such as cancer and heart disease and disorders such as atherosclerosis, stroke, diabetes, and various neurodegenerative diseases such as Alzheimer's and Parkinson's are reduced by antioxidant compounds (Vuksan et al., 2007). The antioxidant activity of hydrolyzed and nonhydrolyzed extract of chia seeds was also evaluated by Miller in 1971 using the oxidation reaction of b-carotene and linoleic acid. Results showed flavanols glycosides as the major antioxidant in the nonhydrolyzed extract followed by chlorogenic acid and caffeic acid. In contrast, caffeic acid is the primary antioxidant source in the hydrolyzed fraction. Industrial uses of chia gum are also very prominent as dietary fibers in foods have physiological functionality for their beneficial effect on human health. The technological functionality of chia seeds greatly depends on the hydration properties of fibers (Borderías et al. 2005). Significant technical/functional properties are water-holding and absorption capacity, solubility and swelling, viscosity, and gelling. Chia is a starting material in the food industry for its dietary fiber content. Gum from chia seeds can be extracted from the dietary fiber of chia by treatment of seeds with water. It can be used to control viscosity, stability, texture, and consistency when added as an additive in food systems (Capitani et al., 2015). The gum is also stable at high temperatures making gum extracted from chia seed a promising agent in high-value food formulations (Timilsena et al., 2016). Segura-Campos et al. (2014) studied the chemical and functional properties of chia seed gum. They reported water-holding (110.5 g/g) as an essential physicochemical characteristic in the food industry. Chia gum was shown to contain 26.5% of fat and, when submitted to fat extraction, produced two fractions: gum with fat (FCG) and gum partially defatted (PDCG) (Segura-Campos et al., 2014). The PDCG has a high protein, appreciable amount of ash, and significant carbohydrate content than the FCG. The functional properties of fatted and defatted chia gum were analyzed that found that lower oil holding ability (11.68 g/g) and water absorption (36.26 g/g) in defatted gum, possess more excellent oil holding (24.89 g/g) and water absorption (44.12 g/g) in fatted gum. The FRF is mainly composed of IDF (94.9%) with only a very minor amount of soluble fiber (5.4%) (Vazquez-Ovando et al., 2009). Scientists also evaluated the other two crucial properties of chia FRF, which were the emulsifying activity. The ability to facilitate the solubilization or dispersion of two immiscible liquids was studied.

Furthermore, the emulsifying stability is the ability to maintain an emulsion (54.16 mL/100 mL and 94.89 mL/100 mL, respectively). It can be, therefore, a valid alternative in foods as a foam stabilizer and emulsifier. Microstructural features of chia seeds were also studied by light and scanning electron microscopy by Munoz et al. (2012). They explained the extraordinary capacity of chia mucilage hydration, reporting water retention of 27 times of its weight, almost double that of those reported by Vazquez-Ovando et al. (2009), in which only the FRF was hydrated. Later on, they produced a mixture of mucilage of *S. hispanica*, and why protein concentrates in proportions 1:3 and 1:4 as a new source of polymer blends to develop coatings and edible films which may be used as a protective water vapor barrier (Munoz et al., 2012). It is also used as such or in whole-seeds as a component of the biodegradable film (Capitani et al., 2016) as a thickening agent for bread and pasta (e.g., Menga et al., 2017), cosmetic use, and medical uses (Vuksan et al., 2010). Recent studies demonstrated that chia seeds have great potential for developing healthy and good-quality meat and fish products. A recent report conducted by Ding et al. (2017) demonstrated that a combination of chia (1%) and carrageenan (0.5%) increases the production yield of restructured ham-like products and decreases lipid and protein oxidation. Chia oil also contributed to an enhancement in the nutritional quality of tilapia fillets, in terms of omega-3 fatty acids content and total antioxidant capacity (Montanher et al., 2016). It has been reported that macerated chia seeds in methanol show an anticorrosion effect on steel mainly attributed to the unsaturated fatty acids (Hermoso-Diaz et al., 2014).

However, more studies are needed to validate their biological effects and confirm the results of scientific investigations to make more conclusive interpretations of the outcomes of chia seed intake and its effects on human health.

BIBLIOGRAPHY

Anderson, J. W., Baird, P., Davis, R. H., Ferreri, S., Knudtson, M., Koraym, A., Williams, C. L. (2009). Health benefits of dietary fiber. *Nutr Rev* 67:188–205.

Ayerza, R. (2013a). Seed composition of two chia (Salvia hispanica L.) genotypes which differ in seed color Emir. *J Food Agric* 25:495–500.

Ayerza, R. (2013b). Composition of chia (Salvia hispanica) grown in six tropical and subtropical ecosystems of South America. *J Food Agric* 25:495–500.

Ayerza, R. and Coates, W. (2004). Composition of chia (Salvia hispanica L.) grown in six tropical and subtropical ecosystems of South America. *Trop Sci* 44:131–135.

Ayerza, h. R., and Coates, W. (2011). Protein content, oil content and fatty acid profiles as potential criteria to determine the origin of commercially grown chia (*Salvia hispanica* L.). *Ind Crop Prod* 34(2):1366–1371. https://doi.org/10.1016/j.indcrop.2010.12.007

Balasundram, N., Sundram, K., and Samman, S. (2006). Phenolic compounds in plants and agri-industrial by-products: antioxidant activity, occurrence and potential uses. *Food Chem* 99:191–203.

Bushway, A. A., Belyea, P. R., and Bushway, R. J. (1981). Chia seed as a source of oil, polysaccharide, and protein. *J Food Sci* 46:1349–1350.

Capitani, M. I., Corzo-Rios, L. J., Chel-Guerrero, L. A., Betancur-Ancona, D. A., Nolasco, S. M., and Tomas M. C. (2015). Rheological properties of aqueous dispersions of chia (Salvia hispanica L.) mucilage. *J Food Eng* 149:70–77.

Capitani, M. I., Spotorno, V., Nolasco, S. M., and Tomas, M. C. (2012). Physicochemical and functional characterization of by-products from chia (*Salvia hispanica* L.) seeds of Argentina. *LWT – Food Sci Technol* 45(1):94–102. https://doi.org/10.1016/j.lwt.2011.07.012

Codex Alimentarius Commission; Food and Agriculture Organization; World Health Organization (2009). Report of the 30th session of the Codex Committee on nutrition and foods for special dietary uses. ALINORM 09/32/26

Cushnie, T. P. T. and Lamb, A. J. (2005). Antimicrobial activity of flavonoids. *Int J Antimicrob Agents* 26:343–356.

Da̧browski, G., Konopka, I., Czaplicki, S., and Tanska, M. (2016). Composition and oxidative stability of oil from Salvia hispanica L. seeds in relation to extraction method. *Eur J Lipid Sci Technol.* doi:10.1002/ejlt.201600209

Ding, Y., Lin, H. W., Lin, Y. L., Yang, D. J., Yu, Y. S., Chen, J. W., Wang, S. Y., and Chen, Y. C. (2017) Nutritional composition in the chia seed and its processing properties on restructured ham-like products. *J Food Drug Anal.* doi:10.1016/j.jfda.2016.12. 012

Hermoso-Diaz, I. A., Velazquez-Gonzalez, M. A., Lucio-Garcia, M. A., Gonzalez-Rodriguez, J. G. (2014). A study of Salvia hispanica as green corrosion inhibitor for carbon steel in sulfuric acid. *Chem Sci Rev Lett* 3:685–697.

Ixtaina, V. Y., Martinez, M. L., Spotorno, V., Mateo, C. M., Maestri, D. M., Diehl, B. W. K., Nolasco, S. M., and Tomas, M. C. (2011). Characterization of chia seed oils obtained by pressing and solvent extraction. *J Food Compos Anal* 24:166–174.

Lairon, D., Arnault, N., Bertrais, S., Planells, R., Clero, E., Hercberg, S., Boutron-Ruault, M. C. (2005). Dietary fiber intake and risk factors for cardiovascular disease in French adults. *Am J Clin Nutr* 82:1185–1194.

Li, B. Q., Fu, T., Dongyan, Y., Mikovits, J. A., Ruscetti, F. W., and Wang, J. M. (2000). Flavonoid baicalin inhibits HIV-1 infection at the level of viral entry. *Biochem Biophys Res Commun* 276(2):534–538.

Lu, Y. and Foo, L. Y. (2002). Polyphenolics of Salvia—a review. *Phytochemistry* 59:117–140.

Matthaus, B. (2002) Antioxidant activity of extracts obtained from residues of different oilseeds. *J Agric Food Chem* 50:3444–3452.

Menga, V., Amato, M., Phillips, T. D., Angelino, D., Morreale, F., and Fares, C. (2017). Gluten-free pasta incorporating chia (Salvia hispanica L.) As thickening agent: an approach to naturally improve the nutritional profile and the in vitro carbohydrate digestibility. *Foog Chem* 221:1954–1961.

Montanher, P. F., Costa e Silva, B., Bonafe, E. G., Carbonera, F., dos Santos, H. M. C., de Lima Figueiredo, I., Maruyama, S. A., Matsushita, M. (2016) Effects of diet supplementation with chia (Salvia hispanica L.) oil and natural antioxidant extract on the omega-3 content and antioxidant capacity of Nile tilapia fillets. *Eur J Lipid Sci Technol* 118:698–707.

Montonen, J., Knekt, P., Jarvinen, R., Aromaa, A., and Reunanen, A. (2003). Whole-grain and fiber intake and the incidence of type 2 diabetes. *Am J Clin Nutr* 77:622–629.

Petruzziello, L., Iacopini, F., Bulajic, M., Shah, S., and Costamagna, G. (2006). Review article: uncomplicated diverticular disease of the colon. *Aliment Pharmcol Ther* 23:1379–1391.

Reyes-Caudillo, E., Tecante, A., and Valdivia-Lopez, M. A. (2008). Dietary fibre content and antioxidant activity of phenolic compounds present in Mexican chia (*Salvia hispanica* L.) seeds. *Food Chem* 107(2):656–663. https://doi.org/10.1016/j.foodchem.2007.08.062

Segura-Campos, M. R., Ciau-Solıs, N., Rosado-Rubio, G., Chel-Guerrero, L., and Betancur-Ancona, D. (2014). Chemical and functional properties of chia seed (*Salvia hispanica* L.) gum. *Int J Food Sci* 2014:1–5. https://doi.org/10.1155/2014/241053

Timilsena, Y. P., Adhikari, R., Barrow, C. J., and Adhikari, B. (2016). Physicochemical and functional properties of protein isolate produced from Australian chia seeds. *Food Chem* 212:648–656. https://doi.org/10.1016/j.foodchem.2016.06.017

Vazquez-Ovando, A., Rosado-Rubio, G., Chel-Guerrero, L., and Betancur-Ancona, D. (2009). Physicochemical properties of a fibrous fraction from chia (Salvia hispanica L.). *LWT—Food Sci Technol* 42:168–217.

Vuksan, V., Whitham, D., Sievenpiper, J. L., Jenkins, A. L., Rogovik, A. L., Bazinet, R. P., et al. (2007). Supplementation of conventional therapy with the novel grain salba (*Salvia hispanica* L.) improves major and emerging cardiovascular risk factors in type 2 diabetes: Results of a randomized controlled trial. *Diabetes Care* 30(11):2804–2810. https://doi.org/10.2337/dc07-1144.

Weber, C. W., Gentry, H. S., Kohlhepp, E. A., and McCrohan, P. R. (1991). The nutritional and chemical evaluation of chia seeds. *Ecol Food Nutr* 26:119–125.

Whelton, S. P., Hyre, A. D., Pedersen, B., Yi Y., Whelton, P. K., and He, J. (2005). Effect of dietary fiber intake on blood pressure: a meta-analysis of randomized, controlled clinical trials. *J Hypertens* 23:475–481.

Yao, L. H., Jiang, Y. M., Shi, J., Tomas-Barberan, F. A., Datta, N., Singanusong, R., and Chen, S. S. (2004). Flavonoids in food and their health benefits. *Plant Food Hum Nutr* 59:113–122.

Zandi, K., Teoh, B. T., Sam, S. S., Wong, P. F., Mustafa, M. R., and Abubakar, S (2011). Antiviral activity of four types of bioflavonoid against dengue virus type-2. *Virol J* 8: 560–571.

Zhu, W., Jia, Q., Wang, Y., Zhang, Y., and Xia, M. (2012). The anthocyanin cyanidin-3-O-b-glucoside, a flavonoid, increases hepatic glutathione synthesis and protects hepatocytes against reactive oxygen species during hyperglycemia: involvement of a cAMP–PKA-dependent signaling pathway. *Free Radical Bio Med* 52:314–327.

4 Quinoa and Chia Seeds for Human Health

Quinoa and chia seeds have gained popularity in recent years. The concept of consuming superfoods as health-promoting factors is on pace, and people are getting interested in their properties. Knowing about quinoa and chia seeds' magnificent characteristics, researchers are also keenly analyzing their potential in the food market. Aztecs and Mayas used chia seeds to prepare various herbal medicines, folk food, and traditional paintings. The seeds of chia, corn, and amaranth were among the main components of the diet of the pre-columbian peoples of America whose diets, when compared with their modern counterparts, surprisingly met the dietary requirements which are established today by the Food and Agriculture Organization and the World Health Organization (FAO, 2011). These seed types were recognized for their nutritional and medicinal properties by the ancient civilizations that inhabited South America (Ayerza and Coates, 2005; Whistler, 1982). Although chia seeds were consumed as a foodstuff in some regions, oil from the seeds was extracted to use for cosmetic purposes. In Communities like Aztecs, chia was used in religious rituals to offer God as a ceremonial gift (Beltrán-Orozco and Romero, 2003; Hentry et al., 1990). There are many theories regarding the name of chia, and most adopted is that the word 'chia' is a Spanish adaptation of chain or Chien, which means 'oily', that comes from Nahuatl. The name was first adopted by Swedish botanical scientist Karl Linnaeus. The former territory of Nahuatl Chiapan, meaning 'River of Chia', took its name from the plant, and on the banks of the Grijalva River, the plant has been grown since ancient times. Today these lands form the Mexican state of Chiapas. The pre-Columbian peoples also used chia to prepare a beverage called 'chia fresca' (fresh chia), consumed even in today's world.

The Spanish trouncing repressed many of the folklores of the pre-Columbian peoples and vanished almost everything of their agricultural production and marketing system. Many of the crops that constituted the daily diet of pre-Columbian America were destroyed because of their close association with religion, to be replaced by foreign species such as wheat, barley, and carrots, which were in great demand among the conquerors (Ayerza and Coates, 2005; Craig, 2004). As mentioned in previous chapters, chia seed is a natural source of omega-3 (α-linolenic acid), high fiber content, proteins of high biological value, and natural antioxidants that protect the seed against certain adverse conditions, in addition to other important nutritional components such as vitamins and minerals (Bushway, 1981; Ayerza, 1995; Ayerza and Coates, 2005). Scientists have since concluded that pre-Columbian diets were, in the primary, nutritionally superior to what people eat today (Ayerza and Coates, 1990).

DOI: 10.1201/9781003080770-4

NUTRITIONAL VALUE

Chia is nowadays classified as a nonconventional seed, as it is not consumed in the regular diets of different countries, but this situation is changing. High concentrations of the essential fatty acid α-linolenic acid (ALA, 18:3 n-3) are found in chia seeds, which are further associated with specific physiological functions (Chicco et al., 2009; Fernandez et al., 2008; Meester et al., 2008). The seed contains significant primary and synergistic natural antioxidants, such as chlorogenic acid, caffeic acid, myricetin, quercetin, and kaempferol (Taga et al., 1984; Ayerza and Coates, 2001; Ayerza and Coates, 2001). Out of the oil in chia seeds, omega-3 has a 75% share as a nutraceutical component (Taga et al., 1984; Ixtaina et al., 2011). With significant amount of dietary fiber, it forms a good replacer of luxatives (Vázquez-Ovando 2009; Capitani et al., 2012). It has been observed that when the seed is placed in an aqueous medium, it exudes a mucilaginous polysaccharide that surrounds the seed (Muñoz, 2012). Salgado-Cruz M, D. C-L, and M. BO, in the year 2005, reported that consumption of chia seed mucilage improves digestion, and with the seed, it constitutes a nutritious food source. Furthermore, the seed contains more protein than any other grain, is gluten-free, and contains no toxic components. Finally, it is an essential source of vitamins and minerals (Table 4.1).

TABLE 4.1
Nutritional Composition of Chia Seed and Other Seeds (per 100 g)

Seed	Chia Seed	Chia Seed	Quinoa Seed	Amaranth	Flaxseed
Reference	USDA (2011)	Ayerza and Coates (2009)	Wright et al. (2002)	Alvarez Jubete et al. (2009)	Morris (2007)
Energy (K cal)	486	n/r	n/r	n/r	450
Protein (g)	16.54	15.95–26.03	14.8–25.7	14.9	20
Total fat (g)	30.74	29.98–33.5	5.3–6.2	9.1	41
Saturated fatty acid (g)	3.33	3.1–3.4	n/r	2.45	n/r
Monounsaturated fatty acid (g)	2.309	n/r	n/r	2.017	n/r
Polyunsaturated fatty acid (g)	23.67	23.6–27.75	n/r	4.47	23
Trans fatty acid (g)	0.14	n/r	n/r	0.02	n/r
Omega-3 fatty acid (g)	17.83	n/r	n/r	n/r	n/r
Cholesterol (mg)	0	n/r	n/r	n/r	0.09
Carbohydrate (g)	42.12	n/r	55.8–69.1	70.3	29
Fiber, total dietary (g)	34.4	n/r	8.8–12.1	12	28

n/r: not reported

FIBER

Dietary fiber in foods, especially whole grains, is a vital biocomponent due to its potential health benefit. Many research studies have shown the effect of fiber consume such as the decrease of risk for coronary heart disease, risk for diabetes mellitus type 2, and several types of cancer (Lattimer and Haub, 2010; Steinmetz and Potter, 1996; Kaczmarczyk et al., 2012). On the other hand, dietary fiber consumption has increased postmeal satiety and decreased subsequent hunger (Archer, 2004; Redgwell and Fischer, 2005). According to the American Dietetic Association (ADA), dietary fiber has demonstrated health maintenance and disease prevention benefits. The recommendation for adult dietary fiber intake generally ranges from 20 to 35 g/day (Marlett, 2002). Chia seeds contain between 35 and 42 g of dietary fiber per 100 g, equivalent to almost 100% of the daily recommendations for the adult population; the defatted flour possesses 40% fiber, 6%–10% of which is soluble and forms form of the mucilage (Bushway, 1981; Reyes-Caudillo, 2008). Interestingly, the fiber content of chia is higher than quinoa, flaxseed, amaranth and even more significant than other dried products (Table 4.2). Therefore, chia seed can be used to prevent many cardiovascular diseases and diabetes, as demonstrated by several epidemiological studies (Ayerza and Coates, 2011; Marlett, 2002; Anderson et al., 1994; Anderson et al., 2009).

LIPIDS AND LIPIDS COMPONENTS

One of the essential characteristics of chia seed is its high content in polyunsaturated fatty acids (Jamboonsri, 2012; Martínez et al., 2012). Table 4.1 shows the composition of saturated, monounsaturated, polyunsaturated, trans, and omega-3 fatty acids. Chia seed contains the highest known percentage of ALA fatty acid of any plant source (Ayerza and Coates, 2011). The fatty acids present in chia have been related to health benefits by numerous authors (Calder and Yaqoob, 2009; Domingo, 2007; Sinn and Howe, 2008; Siegel and Ermilov, 2012). Recent studies by Ciftci et al. (2012) show that chia seed possesses the highest PUFA content, more than 80.5%, and the best ration-6/n-3 compared with flaxseed and perilla contain interesting amounts of tocopherols and sterols (Ciftci et al., 2012). Some studies have shown that ALA can act as a precursor of PUFA; supplementation the diet with high levels of ALA leads to small but significant increases in eicosapentaenoic acid (EPA) and DPA in humans (Harper et al., 2006; Brenna, 2009).

TABLE 4.2
Total Dietary Fiber Content in Foods (%)

Chia	34.4	Plums (dried)	7.1
Flaxseed	27.3	Figs (dried)	9.8
Amaranth	6.7	Apple (dried)	8.7
Quinoa	7.0	Banana (dried)	9.9
Almonds	12.2	Peaches (dried)	8.2
Peanuts	8.5	Pears (dried)	7.5
Soy	9.6		

TABLE 4.3
Protein Content Comparison between Chia Seeds and Cereals

Grain	% of Proteins
Chia	20.70
Oats	16.89
Wheat	13.68
Barley	12.48
Corn	9.42
Rice	6.5

PROTEINS

The protein content of chia seeds varies between 15% and 23% depending on the geographic location of the crop and growing conditions, exceeding that of traditional cereals such as wheat, corn, rice, oats, and barley and other seeds such as amaranth and quinoa (Ayerza and Coates, 2001; Vázquez-Ovando, 2010). Table 4.3 shows the protein content of chia seeds compared to other commonly consumed cereals. The seed does not contain gluten, so celiac disease patients can ingest any food prepared using chia as its basis.

VITAMINS

Chia is prominently a good source of B vitamins (Table 4.4). The seed has much more niacin content than other cereals grains than crops like rice, corn, and soybeans. Consequently, its thiamine and riboflavin content is similar to rice and corn (Beltrán-Orozco and Romero, 2003; Bushway et al., 1981).

MINERALS

Chia is found to be an excellent source of minerals and contains almost six times more calcium, eleven times more phosphorus, and four times more potassium than 100 g of milk, besides magnesium, iron, zinc, and copper(Beltrán-Orozco and Romero, 2003). Chia contains 14–355 times more calcium, 2–11 times more phosphorus, and 1.7–9 times more potassium than 100 g of wheat, rice, oats, and corn. The iron content of chia is also relatively good compared to many other seeds – it has six times more iron than spinach, 1.7 times more than lentils, and 2.5 times more than liver (Beltrán-Orozco and Romero, 2003; Bushway et al., 1981).

ANTIOXIDANTS

Oxidation is an important biological process crucial for energy production in human beings. When electrons are being transferred, free reactive forms of oxygen are generated, such as hydrogen peroxide, hydroxyl, and peroxide radicals. Free radicals

TABLE 4.4
Compositional Analysis of Mineral and Vitamins Present in Quinoa and Chia Seeds (mg/100 g edible portion)

	Quinoa[1]	Chia[2]
Minerals		
Calcium	47	631
Magnesium	197	350
Copper	0.6	1.4
Potassium	563	407
Phosphorus	457	860
Iron	4.6	7.72
Zinc	3.1	4.58
Sodium	5	16
Vitamins		
Thiamin B1	0.36	0.62
Riboflavin B2	0.32	0.17
Niacin B3	1.52	8.82
Folic acid	78.1	–
α-Tocopherol	2.44	–
β-Carotene	8	–

[1] Abeywardena et al. (1991).
[2] Abugoch Ahmed et al. (2006).

are considered the cause of neurological diseases, inflammations, immunodeficiency, aging, ischemic heart disease, strokes, Alzheimer's and Parkinson's diseases, and cancers. The substances like sterols, tocopherols, gallic acids, protocatechuic acid, p-coumaric acids, caffeic acid, chlorogenic acid, epicatechin, quercetin, kaempferol, rutin, and apigenin are found in chia seeds. Chia seed has several compounds that can act as antioxidants, an asset that makes the seed even more attractive. Tocopherols are among the most important phenolic compounds. These compounds are known as primary and synergic antioxidants and make a proportionally greater contribution to the antioxidant activity of chia (Fernández et al., 2006). Total amount of tocopherols in chia seed (239–426 mg/kg) are similar to peanut oil (398.8 mg/kg) but lower than flaxseed (587.5 mg/kg), sunflower (634.7 mg/kg), and soybean (797.5 mg/kg) (Tuberoso et al., 2007). Quercetin and CGA complex are powerful antioxidants with cardioprotective effects (Pandey and Rizvi, 2009).

HUMAN CONSUMPTION

The chia seed is used in countries such as Mexico, Argentina, Chile, New Zealand, Japan, the United States, Canada, and Australia. In 2009, it was approved as a Novel Food by the European Parliament and Council of Europe. It is used as a nutritional supplement ingredient in snacks, biscuits, pasta, yogurt, bread, and even in cake formulations (Company, 2009; Borneo, 2010). Another essential characteristic of this seed is its use in the production of oil. It is light in color and has the advantage of containing essential oils in large numbers. This is also used in making capsules of omega-3 as a nutrient supplement by encapsulation process. Oil extracted from chia leaves can be used as a condiment or fragrance (Beltrán-Orozco and Romero, 2003; Ahmed et al., 1994). Chia seed is one of the most significant natural sources of omega-3, the main effect of which is to reduce triglycerides (Jin et al., 2012), and the presence of phytosterols as β-sitosterol can control cholesterol plasma levels (Alonso-Calderón et al., 2013). Recently, chia seed contains high phytosterols (Ciftci et al., 2012). These essential nutrients help prevent cardiovascular diseases and possess anticancer antioxidants, bactericidal, and antifungal effects (Alonso-Calderón et al., 2013). As discussed above, the seed is rich in dietary fibers and contains highly nutritious proteins, more than traditional cereals (Segura-Campos et al., 2013). It provides an appreciable amount of B vitamins plus minerals such as calcium, magnesium, phosphorus, zinc, potassium, and others (Bushway et al., 1981; USDA, 2011). Another application is using the mucilage of chia in the food industry. This component is composed mainly of polysaccharides in the form of soluble fiber. A recent study demonstrated that mucilage could be a new source of polysaccharides with the potentials of generating different polymer blends to produce films and coatings with improved properties (Muñoz et al., 2012).

PEST CONTROL

In the case of chia, an essential oil can be extracted from the leaves containing components like β-caryophyllene; globulol; γ-muroleno; β-pinene; α-humoleno; germacren-B, and widdrol, and these have a repellent effect against insects (Pascual-Villalobos, 1997; Ahmed et al., 1994).

MEDICINAL USES

Some of the most critical medical studies related to chia have been carried out at the St. Michael Hospital in Toronto, Canada (Vuksan et al., 2007; Vuksan et al., 2010). Chia is rich in soluble fiber. Only 12 g of seed provides more than 5 g of dietary fiber. The insoluble fiber can absorb a good amount of water, which helps in providing a feeling of fullness and slows the digestion process, leading to a stable increase in blood sugar levels and a more stable insulin release. Research carried out by Vuksan et al. in 2007 suggested that a high-fiber diet may be proven helpful in controlling diabetes. The study was conducted on 20 diabetic patients given bread made with chia flour and other whole chia seeds to be sprinkled on foods at home. Results of the study showed the most important findings – blood became less prone to coagulation, blood glucose level decreased, decreased levels of internal inflammation as measured by C-reactive protein (CRP). Chia affected blood pressure. Also, various studies (Fernandez et al., 2008; Ayerza and Coates, 2001; Ayerza and Coates, 2001) have attributed the following medicinal properties to the seed – reduce cholesterol, inhibits blood clotting and promotes tissue regeneration, reduce the digestion time of carbohydrates, assisting in the control of blood sugar levels, decrease the risk of brain diseases, depression, and epilepsy, improves the immune system. Several clinical and epidemiological studies propose that higher consumption of ALA reduces the risk of cardiovascular diseases (EFSA, 2005; Brouwer et al., 2004; Lemaitre et al., 2003; Djoussé et al., 2005).

On the other hand, a study to assess the effectiveness of chia in weight loss and altering disease risk factors in overweight adults found that chia seed increased plasma ALA concentrations. However, no changes were observed in the placebo and chia groups in EPA, docosapentaenoic acid (DHA) concentrations, body composition, inflammation, oxidative stress, and blood pressure. Moreover, in a study done in postmenopausal women ingesting 25 g/day milled chia seed during 7 weeks, plasma ALA, EPA increased significantly after 1-week supplementation. However, no significant changes in plasma DPA and DHA were observed by Jin et al. (2012). According to Mohd Ali et al. (2012), the differences observed in the few clinical studies conducted to date on the seed, mainly the negative results showed by Nieman (2009), may be due to the treatment period used and the components used to each study.

QUINOA SEEDS

The socioeconomic changes such as rising income due to increased urbanization have recognized the role of crops that contribute a high amount of proteins in a healthy human diet (Henchion et al., 2017). The annual global protein demand for approximately 7.3 billion people worldwide is approximately 202 million tonnes (Alonso Miravalles and O'Mahony, 2018; Kim et al., 2019). Animal proteins have high nutritional values, negatively impacting the environment – the increased consumption of animal protein results in concerns for sustainability and food security.

Moreover, it negatively affects greenhouse gas emissions, biodiversity, and other essential ecosystem services (Henchion et al., 2017). Plant-based protein ingredients are getting more popular due to their contribution to environmental sustainability and their cost-effectiveness and food security issues compared with animal-based proteins (Aiking, 2011). The plant-based protein is obtained mainly from seeds, grains, legumes, leaves, etc. Pseudocereals such as amaranth, quinoa, buckwheat, and chia seeds are consumed with greater acceptance due to their high essential amino acid content and various other nutrients present in them (de Frutos et al., 2019). They are easily digestible with an adequate amount of essential amino acids and are effective against several diseases (Mir et al., 2019). Quinoa seeds are rich in nutrients like fatty acids, dietary fiber, protein, essential amino acids, vitamins, antioxidants, and minerals like phosphorus, manganese, calcium, potassium, and sodium. It can be considered a superfood with the highest sources of omega-3 fatty acids and a good quantity of proteins present in it.

Quinoa seed contains all amino acids essential for the human body in their day-to-day life. The essential amino acids required for human nutrition are isoleucine, leucine, lysine, methionine, phenylalanine, threonine, tryptophan, histidine, and valine (SandovalOliveros and Paredes-López, 2013). Glutamic acid is the highest present among all amino acids, and histidine is the least present in quinoa and chia seeds. Quinoa protein demonstrated a quality similar to casein and other milk proteins for quinoa protein (Kozioł, 1992; VegaGálvez et al., 2010). Quinoa has become a significant source of leucine, isoleucine, phenylalanine, glutamic acid, aspartic acid, and tyrosine (Abugoch James, 2009). Quinoa proteins are high in lysine (2.6–7.9 g/100g protein), methionine (0.5–9.6 g/100g protein), and threonine (2.2–8.4 g/ 100g protein), which are the deficient amino acids in conventional cereals, such as wheat and maize (Dini et al., 2005). The protein quality also depends on protein digestibility, the influence of antinutritional factors, and the ratio between tryptophan and neutral amino acids (Comai et al., 2007).

NUTRITION AND HEALTH BENEFITS

Quinoa seed is rich in nutrients than many other vegetable sources. Its amino acid composition is close to the ideal protein equilibrium recommended by the FAO and similar to milk. It possesses a relatively high level of vitamins and minerals, and lipids on this seed have high quality as edible vegetable oil (Chauhan et al., 1992; Ogungbenle, 2003; Comai et al., 2007; Spehar, 2007; Abugoch James, 2009; Vega-Gálvez et al., 2010). It is also rich in copper, iron, and potassium and provides fiber, vitamin E, magnesium, and some B vitamins and zinc.

Various factors make quinoa appealing for the production system, including the characteristics of the grain and the plant. This grassy crop is an essential source of nourishment for both humans and animals in the Andean region. Proteins, minerals, vitamins, and fibers are found in excellent quantity in the leaves and panicles, and these nutrients also provide good digestibility. The leaves can be consumed in cooking the same way as spinach and flower buttons like broccoli or cabbage flower (Spehar, 2007). The quinoa grain is a starchy raw material with high carbohydrates, consisting mainly of starch and a small percentage of sugars, vitamins of complex B, vitamin E, and C, and minerals like zinc, iron, magnesium, potassium, phosphorus, manganese, copper, and sodium. It contains much higher levels of total protein, methionine, and lysine when compared to traditional cereals such as rice, maize, barley, and wheat, with fatty acids similar to those of soybean oil in its lipid composition (Chauhan et al., 1992; Ogungbenle, 2003; Spehar, 2007; Abugoch James, 2009; Vega-Gálvez et al., 2010). Cereal crops play an important role in human nutrition, contributing approximately to half the energy and protein intake of the population, with wheat, corn, rice, barley, oats, rye, and sorghum being the most important worldwide. When we compare the nutritional components of the cereals with quinoa, we can notice the richness of this crop's nutrients, which contains higher protein, fat, and ash content (USDA, 2011). The total dietary fiber is close to the value found in cereals (7%–9.7% dm), wherein the embryo contains higher levels than those in perisperm. Different studies in individuals with celiac disease showed that the glycemic index of quinoa was slightly lower than that in gluten-free pasta and bread.

Furthermore, quinoa induced levels of free fatty acids were lower than gluten-free pasta, and triglyceride levels were significantly lower than gluten-free bread (Berti et al., 2004). The digestibility of proteins or the bioavailability (true digestibility) of amino acids in quinoa varies according to the variety and treatment that the grains receive, increasing considerably with cooking (Koziol, 1992; Comai et al., 2007; Alves et al., 2008; Abugoch James, 2009). Moreover, it presents a high rate of nonprotein tryptophan, which is more easily absorbed and can increase the availability of this amino acid in the brain, thereby influencing the synthesis of the serotonin neurotransmitter (Comai et al., 2007).

The fatty acid profile of quinoa is similar to corn and soybean oil (Koziol, 1992; Oshodi et al., 1999; Youdim et al., 2000). Essential fatty acids are essential acids, like linoleic and linolenic acids, necessary substrates in animal metabolism. As indicated by the high iodine value (82.7%) observed by Repo-Carrasco et al. (2003), the fatty acids of quinoa oil are polyunsaturated.

Polyunsaturated Fatty Acids have several positive effects on cardiovascular diseases (Abeywardena et al., 1991; Keys and Parlin, 1966) and improve insulin sensitivity.

The chemical stability of the lipids in quinoa flour was studied by Ng et al. (2007), who found that the lipids were stable during 30 days. This stability is due to vitamin E present naturally.

According to their solubility, they are divided into two groups – water-soluble and fat-soluble. Traditionally, they are among the most widely applied chemicals to improve the nutritional value of food products (Mahan and Escott-Stump, 2010; Vega-Gálvez et al., 2010). It has significant concentrations of pyridoxine (B6) and folic acid, whose values of 100 g can meet the needs of children and adults. The contents in 100 g of riboflavin contribute to 80% of children's daily needs and 40% of adults, as cited by Abugoch James (2009). The niacin content does not meet daily needs, but it is an essential source for the diet. The values of thiamine (B1) are lower than those of oats or barley, but riboflavin (B2), pyridoxine (B6), and folic acid are higher than most cereals such as wheat, oats, barley, rye, rice, and maize. Furthermore, quinoa is an excellent source of vitamin E, higher than wheat, as previously described (Rules and Nair, 1993; Abugoch James, 2009; Alvarez-Jubete et al., 2010). Koziol (1992) compared the levels of vitamins in quinoa with some grain and reported that the grain contains substantially more riboflavin, α-tocopherol, β-carotene, and ascorbic acid than rice, barley, and wheat. RepoCarrasco et al. (2003) also reported that quinoa is rich in vitamins A, B2, and E.

Gluten-free cereals and pseudocereals are becoming increasingly important in our day-to-day life. Consumption of these cereals and pseudocereals helps boost our health. Our body needs regular exercise, which gives us physical and mental fitness, and a properly balanced diet that provides us all nutrients essential for our body. So exercise along with a properly balanced diet is the best way for healthy living. Pseudocereals consumption has been associated with a broad spectrum of beneficial effects beyond its mere nutritional value; digestibility, available lysine, net nutrient utilization, and efficiency ratio are other parameters that help better estimate the nutritional value of gluten-free cereals and pseudocereals.

APPLICATION

Quinoa and chia seeds have wide applications in the food industry due to their high nutrient content, beneficial for human health. Chia can be added to white bread as seed and as a source of bioactive peptides (i.e., functional ingredients) to improve its nutritional quality. Chia seed is used for different purposes as a nutritional supplement and as an ingredient in cereal bars, biscuits, pasta, bread, snacks, and yogurt (Borneo et al., 2010). It is used as healthy cooking oil by humans in their diet (Mohd Ali et al., 2012). Chia seed gum was used for food and industrial applications to improve the product's physical parameters like viscosity, stability, texture, and consistency due to its good functional properties (Capitani et al., 2013). Chia plant contained essential oils that can be extracted from the leaves with main components like βcaryophyllene, globulol, γ-muroleno, β-pinene, α-humulene, and windrow that can act as a repellent against insects (Mohd Ali et al., 2012). Chia mucilage was potentially used in the food industries as it contains excellent stabilizing and thickening abilities. Quinoa can be eaten as a rice replacement, or its seeds can even be popped like popcorn (Valencia-Chamorro, 2003). Quinoa flour is consumed by adding a broad range of pastries such as bread, pasta, pancakes, biscuits, noodles, cakes, and crackers. It is also used by being fermented with millet to produce beer-like beverages (Demir, 2014).

USES CHIA AND QUINOA SEEDS IN COMMERCIAL PRODUCTS

Water holding, absorption, and emulsion capacity are significant features in bakery products with good textural properties. Compared with other fiber sources such as soybean, wheat, maize, wheat hulls, the fiber-rich fraction in chia has higher water-holding, absorption, and organic-molecule absorption with high emulsifying activity (53.26 mL/100 mL) and emulsion stability (94.84 mL/100 mL). For this reason, chia can be used in bread, sweets, and cookies (Bresson et al., 2009; Capitani et al., 2012; Alfredo et al., 2009). The bread enriched with chia seeds is important because it increases satiety and alleviates and serves as a prebiotic because of the high pulp content. Bakery products with chia flour can use in diabetic and obese individuals due to low carbohydrate, high protein, and insoluble fiber contents. Celiac patients, due to being gluten-free, can also consume it.

Inglett et al. reported that the use of chia seed-whole oat flour mixture and chia seed-oat bran instead of wheat flour did not affect the structural quality of cookies. Furthermore, chia-oat applications can contribute to developing the nutritional value of various cookies and other bakery products (Inglett GE et al. 2014). One study stated that the fat used in cake making was changed up to 25% with chia mucilage. The nutritional content, basic functional properties, and sensory properties of the cakes were preserved. Chia mucilage could be used as a fat replacer in foods (Bornea et al., 2010; Felisberto et al., 2015). A study in which two types of broth were produced by adding 7.8% chia flour – 0.9% fat and 11% chia flour – 1% fat showed that chia seeds reduced the dimension of bread in both. It is assumed that the reason for this is that dimension of bread does not increase during the fermentation processes because chia seed is gluten-free and interaction between wheat flour proteins (gliadin and glutenin) and chia fiber.

Furthermore, chia flour increased the amount of ash, pulp, and lipid while reducing carbohydrates. The same study emphasized that a broth produced by adding 11% chia could be defined as a functional food due to high dietary fiber content (Coelho and Salas-Mellado, 2015). The effects of chia on the sensory properties of foods have also been studied in many studies. In a study of taste, 90% of the panelists who were evaluating the bread with chia seeds decided that they were either 'relatively lover' or 'very lover', and 83% of panelists stated that they could purchase this product (Coelho and Salas-Mellado 2015). The European Commission limits chia seeds in bread production to 5% (Mohd Ali et al. 2012).

USE IN ANIMAL PRODUCTS

Using structural emulsions as an animal fat replacer, especially olive oil/chia oil emulsions, is considered suitable for producing and developing healthy meat products due to their technological properties and a healthy lipid source (Herrero et al. 2017). Furthermore, studies have shown that chia oil and its by-products can also be used in animal feed industries to obtain animal products enriched with polyunsaturated fatty acids (Coates and Ayerza, 2009). It was determined that sausages produced by adding chia seed had higher protein content than the control group, and there was no difference in fat content. Stickiness and elasticity were found to be lower in the group to which chia was added, but hardness and chewiness were found to be higher than in the group to which lard was added (Herrero et al., 2017). Another study using chia emulsion as a fat replacer in sausages emphasized that sausages can be accepted despite differences in sensory properties (Pintado et al., 2010). A study was carried out by adding carrageenan and chia and animal fat to ham-like products. It was determined that adding 0.5% carrageenan and 1.0% chia seed was similar to ham-like products 5% lard. Generally, it has been emphasized that chia has improved physicochemical and sensory properties and positively affected the nutritional value of ham-like products. It has also been reported that the polyphenols in chia may partly contribute to the shelf life of these ham-like products (Ding et al., 2018). Some investigations on the effects of chia seed on animal foods have revealed that egg and pig meat increase n-3 quantities, and customer likings have not changed in the worst (Coates and Ayerza 2009). A study using flaxseed, rapeseed, and chia seed as a chicken feed emphasized that the eggs of chia-fed chickens had the highest content of α-linolenic acid compared to chickens fed with linseed or rape (Antruejo et al., 2011). There was no difference between egg weight, egg yolk weight, cholesterol levels, and albumin levels in a study in which eggs were fed with flaxseed and chia seeds at different rates for 30 days. The addition of flaxseed and chia seed increased the amount of α-linolenic acid while the amount of arachidonic acid and polyunsaturated fatty acids decreased. The ratio of n-6/n-3 and saturated fat/n-3 decreased as the amount of chia seed increased (Ayerza and Coates, 2001). Ayerza and Coates found that 280 g/kg of chia seed caused an increase in egg yield of brown chickens without any adverse effects. The same situation was observed in white chickens with 70 g/kg of chia seed (Ayerza and Coates, 2002). In the meat of pigs and rabbits fed with chia seed, the content of polyunsaturated fatty acids increased in meat oils and aroma and flavor (Coates and Ayerza, 2009; Masoero et al., 2008; Dalle Zotte and Szendro, 2011). In a study on rabbits fed with a diet consisting of 0%, 10%, 15% of chia seed, it was emphasized that the content of α-linolenic acid in rabbits fed with a diet containing 10% and 15% of chia seed increased by 20.9% and 25.2%, respectively, compared to the control group and decreased atherogenic and thrombogenic indices (Peiretti and Meineri,

2008). A study of chia-fed chickens reported that αlinolenic acid content of light and dark-colored meat increased. In contrast, saturated fat content and the animal body mass decreased (Ayerza et al., 2002).

In Europe, the chia seed oil is also used in sports drinks, cornflakes, and chocolate other than bakery and meat products [https://www.cbi.eu/market-information/oilseeds/chia-seeds/europe/ (Accessed 2017-08-01)]. It is envisaged that chia seed can be used in commercial marmalades and sauces since the gelling properties of chia seed are very close to the modified pectin species. A study conducted by adding 5% chia seed to strawberry marmalade found that phenolic components and diet fiber increased 15.45% and 168%, respectively, and energy value decreased 48%. At the end of the study, it is stated that strawberry marmalade with chia seed-added and sugar-free strawberry marmalade can be considered a new functional food because of its high antioxidant, dietary fiber, and n-3 values (Ozbek, 2016). A study realized that adding chia protein hydrolysates to carrot cream was 17.52–18.88 mmol/L-mg in the group with chia protein hydrolysates.

In comparison, antioxidant activity was 10.21 mmol/L-mg in the control group (Segura-Campos et al., 2013). Campos et al. have used chia mucilage as an emulsifier and stabilizer in ice cream production. They have found positive effects on the quality of products other than dark color (Campas et al., 2016).

USE IN MICROENCAPSULATION

Chia seeds are highly susceptible to oxidation as they contain significant amounts of polyunsaturated fatty acids. Therefore, effective encapsulation is required to protect them from oxidative degradation during production and storage (Timilsena et al., 2017). The contents of chia's linoleic acid and α-linolenic acid cause poor oxidative stability and shorter shelf life. However, these fatty acids are favorable in terms of nutrition (Martinez et al., 2015). In a study comparing the oxidative stability of chia and walnut oil, this value was 2.88 ± 0.22 hours for walnut oil. In comparison, the oxidative stability index for chia oil was 1.14 ± 0.10 hours (Martinez et al., 2015). In another study, the oxidative stability index of chia was found to be 2.4 hours, which is lower than the oxidative stability index values of canola (12–17 hours), olive (6–11 hours), and coconut oil (33 hours) (Timilsena et al., 2017). The microencapsulation technique affects the oxidative stability of chia oil positively. Chia oil has much more oxidative damage than microencapsulated chia oil during storage (Martinez et al., 2015). In a study, mucilage and soluble proteins extracted from chia and flaxseed encapsulated probiotic bacteria such as *Bifidobacterium infantis* and *Lactobacillus plantarum*. The survivability and viability of these probiotics were assessed after spray drying and during storage. *B. infantis* and *L. plantarum* survived at high rates after encapsulation (98%), and researchers concluded that encapsulation with chia could increase the resistance of probiotics to gastric juice and bile acid. The encapsulated probiotics added to the juice show high activity after storage for 45 days at 4°C (Bustamante et al., 2017). A study comparing the release of encapsulated and unencapsulated chia oil during oral, gastric, and intestinal digestive steps has determined that most oil fractions (38%–84% of the initial volume) are released in the gastric phase. In contrast, less is released in the intestinal phase

(Timilsena et al., 2017). The microencapsulation with chia seed protein isolate and chia seed gum resulted in a significant decrease in moisture content and water activity (Timilsena et al., 2016).

Nowadays, scientists have focused on developing edible and biodegradable films as an alternative to synthetic polymers due to environmental problems. Hydrocolloids of chia mucilage are an exciting component for edible film production (Dick et al., 2015). It is thought that these films can increase protection in packaged products by having high water solubility, good thermal resistance, transparency, and is a barrier against UV lights (Dick et al., 2015).

Quinoa-based extruded products developed during recent years can be noted as new quinoa food products. Quinoa products are obtained through the extraction of compounds from quinoa and for the creation of added-value products. Examples of these products will be discussed in detail in Chapter 8. One main product, quinoa, can produce protein concentrate. Compared to the starch content of wheat and barley, quinoa starch shows higher viscosity, higher water retention, expansion capabilities, and higher gelatinization temperatures, resulting in a better performance thickening agent. Quinoa is used in the production of edible films based on its protein and starch content. It may be used as an emulsion stabilizer agent, namely for Pickering emulsions (Wang and Zhu 2016). Quinoa may be incorporated into food products to help extend shelf life and reduce microbial spoilage. The increase in the shelf life of quinoa incorporated food products at the compositional and organoleptic level could be due to the lower rate of degradation in starch molecules. Bioactive components of quinoa inhibits mold growth in food products (Tanwar et al., 2019).

BIBLIOGRAPHY

Abeywardena, M., McLeannan, P., and Charnock, J. (1991). Differential effects of dietary fish oil on myocardial prostaglandin 12 and thromboxane A2 production. *Am J Physiol* 260:379–385.

Abugoch Ahmed, M., Hamed, R., Ali, M., Hassan, A., and Babiker, E. (2006). Proximate composition, antinutritional factors and protein fractions of guar gum seeds as influenced by processing treatments. *Pak J Nutr* 5(5):340–345.

Abugoch James, L. E. (2009). Quinoa (*Chenopodiumquinoa* Willd.): Composition, chemistry, nutritional and functional properties. *Adv Food Nutr Res* 58(cap.1). https://doi.org/10.1016/S1043-4526(09)58001-1

Ahmed, M., Ting, I. P., and Scora, R. W. (1994). Leaf oil composition of *Salvia hispanica* L. from three geographical areas. *J Essent Oil Res* 6(3):223–228.

Aiking, H. (2011). Future protein supply. *Trends Food Sci Technol* 22(2–3):112–120.

Alonso-Calderón, A., Chávez-Bravo, E., Rivera, A., Montalvo-Paquini, C., Arroyo-Tapia, R., Monterrosas-Santamaria, M., Jiménez-Salgado, T., and, Tapia-Hernández, A. (2013). Characterization of black chia seed (Salvia hispanica L.) and oil and quantification of β-sitosterol. International Research *Journal of Biological Sciences* 2(1): 70–72.

Alonso-Miravalles, L. and O'Mahony, J. A. (2018). Composition, protein profile and rheological properties of pseudocereal-based protein-rich ingredients. *Foods* 7(5):73.

Alvarez-Jubete, L., Arendt, E. K., and Gallagher, E. (2010). Nutritive value of pseudocereals and their increasing use as functional gluten-free ingredients. *Trends in Food Science & Technology*, 21(2):106–113.

Alves, L. F., Rocha, M. S., and Gomes, C. C. F. (2008). Avaliação da qualidadeproteica daQuinua Real (*Chenopodiumquinoa* Willd) através de métodosbiológicos. *e-scientia* 1(1):16p.

Ayerza, R. (1995). Oil content and fatty acid composition of chia (Salvia hispanica L.), from five northeastern locations in northwestern Argentina. *J Am Oil Chem Soc* 72:1079–1081.

Ayerza, R. and Coates, W. (2009). Influence of environment on growing period and yield, protein, oil and -linolenic content of three chia (Salvia hispanica L.) selections, *Industrial Crops and Products* 30(2):321–324.

Berti, C., Riso, P., Monti, L. D., and Porrini, M. (2004). In vitro starch digestibility and in vivo glucose response of gluten-free foods and their gluten counterparts. *Eur J Nutr* 43(4):198–204.

Borneo, R., Aguirre, A., and Leon, A. E. (2010). Chia (*Salvia hispanica* L) gel can be used as egg or oil replacer in cake formulations. *J Am Diet Assoc* 110:946–949.

Brouwer, I. A., Katan, M. B., and Zock, P. L. (2004). Dietary α-linolenic acid is associated with reduced risk of fatal coronary heart disease, but increased prostate cancer risk: A meta-analysis. *J Nutr* 134(4):919–922.

Campos, B. E., Ruivo, T. D., Scapim, M. R. S., Madrona, G. S., and Bergamasco, R. C. (2016). Optimization of the mucilage extraction process from chia seeds and application in ice cream as a stabilizer and emulsifier. *LWT - Food Sci Technol* 65:874–883.

Chauhan, G. S., Eskin, N. A. M., and Tkachuk, R. (1992a). Nutrients and antinutrients in quinoa seed. *Cereal Chem* 69:85–88.

Chauhan, G. S., Zillman, R. R., and Eskin, N. A. M. (1992b). Dough mixing and breadmaking properties of quinoa-wheat flour blends. *Int J Food Sci Technol* 27:701–705.

Comai, S., Bertazzo, A., Bailoni, L., Zancato, M., Costa, C. V. L., and Allegri, G. (2007). The content of proteic and nonproteic (free and protein-bound) tryptophan in quinoa and cereal flours. *Food Chem* 100(4):1350–1355. https://doi.org/10.1016/j.foodchem.2005.10.072

deFrutos, M. F., Fotschki, B., Musoles, R. F., and Llopis, J. M. L. (2019). *Gluten-free cereals and pseudocereals: Nutrition and health.* https://doi.org/10.1007/978-3-319-78030-6_60

Demir, M. K. (2014). Use of quinoa flour in the production of gluten-free tarhana. *Food Sci Technol Res.* https://doi.org/10.3136/fstr.20.1087

Djoussé, L., Arnett, D. K., Pankow, J. S., Hopkins, P. N., Province, M. A., and Ellison, R. C. (2005). Dietary linolenic acid is associated with a lower prevalence of hypertension in the NHLBI family heart study. *Hypertension* 45(3):368–373.

EFSA (2005). Opinion of the scientific panel on dietetic products, nutrition and allergies on a request from the Commission related to the safety of chia (*Salvia hispanica L.*) seed and ground whole chia seed as a novel food ingredient intended for use in bread. *EFSA J* 278:1–12.

Fernandez, I. R., Ayerza, W., Coates, S. M., Vidueiros, N. C., Pallaro, A. N. (2006a). Nutritional characteristics of chia. *Actualización en Nutrición* 7:23–25.

Fernandez, I., Vidueiros, S. M., Ayerza, R., Coates, W., and Pallaro, A. (2008). Impact of chia (Salvia hispanica L.) on the immune system: preliminary study. *Proc Nutr Soc* 67:E12 doi:10.1017/S0029665108006216

Henchion, M., Hayes, M., Mullen, A. M., Fenelon, M., & Tiwari, B. (2017). Future protein supply and demand: strategies and factors influencing a sustainable equilibrium. *Foods* 6(7):53.

Keys, A. and Parlin, R. (1966). Serum-cholesterol response to changes in dietary lipids. *Am J Clin Nutr* 19:175–181.

Kim, S. W., Less, J. F., Wang, L., Yan, T., Kiron, V., Kaushik, S. J., and Lei, X. G. (2019). Meeting global feed protein demand: Challenge, opportunity, and strategy. *Annu Rev Anim Biosci.* https://doi.org/10.1146/annurev-animal-030117-014838

Koziol, M. J. (1992). Chemical composition and nutritional evaluation of Quinoa (*Chenopodiumquinoa* Willd.). *J Food Compos Anal.* 5(1):35–68. https://doi.org/10.1016/0889-1575(92)90006-6

Lemaitre, R. N., King, I. B., Mozaffarian, D., Kuller, L. H., Tracy, R. P., and Siscovick, D. S. (2003). n–3 Polyunsaturated fatty acids, fatal ischemic heart disease, and nonfatal myocardial infarction in older adults: The cardiovascular health study. *The Am J Clin Nutr* 77(2):319–325.

Mahan, L.K. and Escott-Stump, S. (2010). *Krause: Alimentos, nutrição e dietoterapia.* 12th ed. Elsevier, Rio de Janeiro, 1351p.

Mir, N. A., Riar, C. S., and Singh, S. (2019). Effect of pH and holding time on the characteristics of protein isolates from Chenopodium seeds and study of their amino acid profile and scoring. *Food Chem.* https://doi.org/10.1016/j.foodchem.2018.08.048

Morris, Diane H. (2007). Flax – A Health and Nutrition Primer Fourth Edition. Flax council of Canada, Figure 2 chapter 2, p. 24

Ng, S., Anderson, A., Cokera, J., and Ondrusa, M. (2007). Characterization of lipid oxidation products in quinoa (Chenopodiumquinoa). *Food Chem* 101(1):185–192.

Nieman, D. C., Cayea, E. J., Austin, M. D., Henson, D. A., McAnulty, S. R., and Jin, F. (2009). Chia seed does not promote weight loss or alter disease risk factors in overweight adults. *Nutr Res* 29:414–418.

Ogungbenle, N. H. (2003). Nutritional evaluation and functional properties of quinoa (Chenopodiumquinoa) flour. *Int J Food Sci Nutr* 54(2):153–158.

Oshodi, A., Ogungbenle, H., and Oladimeji, M. (1999). Chemical composition, nutritionally valuable minerals and functional properties of benniseed, pearl millet and quinoa flours. *Int J Food Sci Nutr* 50:325–331.

Ozbek, T. (2016). Ciyatohumuilaveli, şekerilavesizcilekmarmeladı. PhD dissertation. Istanbul Technical University.

Pandey, K. B. and Rizvi, S. I. (2009). Plant polyphenols as dietary antioxidants in human health and disease. *Oxid Med Cell Longev* 2(5):270–278.

Pascual-Villalobos, M., Correal, E., Molina, E., and Martínez, J. (1997). *Evaluación y selección de especiesvegetalesproductoras de compuestosnaturales con actividadinsecticida.* Centro de Investigación y DesarrolloAgroalimentario (CIDA), Murcia, España.

Repo-Carrasco, R., Espinoza, C., and Jacobsen, S. (2003). Nutritional value and use of the Andean crops quinoa (Chenopodiumquinoa) and kañiwa (Chenopodiumpallidicaule). *Food Rev Int* 19:179–189.

Ruales, J. and Nair, B. M. (1993). Saponins, phytic acid, tannis and protease inhibitors inquinoa (*Chenopodiumquinoa* Willd) seeds. *Food Chem* 48(2):137–143.

Sandoval-Oliveros, M. R. and Paredes-López, O. (2013). Isolation and characterization of proteins from chia seeds (Salvia hispanica L.). *J Agri Food Chem.* https://doi.org/10.1021/jf3034978

Spehar, C. R. (2007). *Quinoa: alternativapara a diversificaçãoagrícola e alimentar.* Ed. Técnico. Embrapa Cerrados, Planaltina, 103p.

The Chia Company (2009). *Request for scientific evaluation of substantial equivalence application for the approval of chia seeds (Salvia Hispanica L.) from The Chia Company for use in bread.* Food Standards Agency, London.

Valencia-Chamorro, S. A. (2003). QUINOA. In *Encyclopedia of food sciences and nutrition.* https://doi.org/10.1016/b0-12-227055-x/00995-0

Vega-Gálvez, A. V., Miranda, M., Vergara, J., Uribe, E., Puente, L., and Martínez, E. A. (2010). Nutrition facts and functional potential of quinoa (Chenopodium quinoa willd.), an ancient Andean grain: A review. *J Sci Food Agri* 90:2541–2547.

Vuksan, V., Jenkins, A. L., Dias, A. G., Lee, A. S., Jovanovski, E., Rogovik, A. L., and Hanna, A. (2010). Reduction in postprandial glucose excursion and prolongation of satiety: possible explanation of the long-term effects of whole grain Salba (*Salvia hispanica* L.). *Eur J Clin Nutr* 64:436–438.

Vuksan, V., Whitham, D., Sievenpiper, J. L., Jenkins, A. L., Rogovik, A. L., Bazinet, R. P., Vidgen, E., and Hanna, A. (2007). Supplementation of conventional therapy with the novel grain Salba (Salvia hispanica L.) improves major and emerging cardiovascular risk factors in type 2 diabetes. *Diabetes Care* 30:2804–2810.

Wright, K. H., Huber, K. C., Fairbanks, D. J., and Huber, C. S. (2002). Isolation and characterization of Atriplex hortensis and sweet Chenopodium quinoa starches. *Cereal Chemistry*, 79, 715–719.

Youdim, K., Martin, A.,s and Joseph, J. (2000). Essential fatty acids and the brain: Possible health implications. *Int J Dev Neurosci* 18(4–5):383–399.

5 *Chenopodium* and *Salvia* as Functional Foods

INTRODUCTION

Quinoa (*Chenopodium quinoa* L.) and chia (*Salvia hispanica* L.) are two plants with unique functional and bioactive characteristics in their seeds and leaves. They are excellent functional grains against physiological diseases such as diabetes, hypertension, cardiovascular diseases, and obesity because they have much greater nutrients and bioactive components (Rendón-Villalobos et al., 2018).

C. quinoa and *Chenopodium album* are a leafy vegetable with grains. *C. album* is a leafy part, and *C. quinoa* is a grain part of green leafy vegetable belongs to the Chenopodiaceae family. It is a Western Asian natural plant and summer annual weed that grows up to 1 m tall. It is primarily grown in western Rajasthan, the Kulu Valley, and Shimla in India. The entire plant is coated in various quantities of waxy material, giving it a light green color. It grows as a weed in wheat or other crops and is used in almost all parts in the form of Sag and Bathua Roti and Bathua Parantha (GuhaBakshi et al., 1999). Various studies have confirmed that the plant and its components are found to be helpful in dealing with anorexia, cough, dysentery, diarrhea, and piles, and tiny worms.

It has also been widely produced for decades as a leafy vegetable and a valuable secondary grain crop for human and animal consumption. It has a high-protein and a well-balanced amino acid spectrum, with high levels of lysine (5.1%–6.4%) and methionine (0.4%–1.0%), and it has vitamin (A, C, and E) and varieties of minerals (Bhargava et al., 2003; Prakash and Pal, 1998). *C. album* is classified as a functional food grain because it contains antioxidants in the form of total phenols and flavonoid glycosides (quercetin, rutin, kaempferol) (Chludil et al., 2008).

Chia seeds, also known as *S. hispanica* L., are species of the Lamiaceae (mint) family. It is a summer-flowering annual plant found in Mexico and Northern Guatemala (Capitani et al., 2012). From ancient times, this chia seed has been famous for its medicinal and nutritional benefits. As chia seeds are taken consumed because of their rich omega-3 fatty acid content, but chia oil was utilized only in cosmetics and paintings (Ayerza & Coates, 2005). Also, chia seeds are considered a good source of polyunsaturated fatty acids (PUFAs, up to 83% of extracted oil), dietary fiber (34.4 g/100 g), total protein (16.54 g/100 g), minerals, and natural antioxidants (Giaretta et al., 2018).

There are many studies on chia and quinoa seed replacement as functional additives in food systems that focus on the nutritional and sensory characterization of the food products (Coorey et al., 2012).

DOI: 10.1201/9781003080770-5

NUTRITIONAL COMPOSITIONS

C. quinoa L. has a large amount of good quality protein so that quinoa seeds are a complete meal with a high nutritional value. Beyond their protein composition, lipids, carbohydrates, minerals, and saponin have all been studied extensively. Furthermore, it also contains vitamins and minerals such as vitamin B, vitamin C, and vitamin E (Oshodi et al., 1999; Koziol, 1993; Chauhan et al., 1992).

S. hispanica L. contains 25%–41% carbohydrate, 20%–22% protein, 30%–35% fat, and 4%–6% ash in terms of macronutrients. Chia seeds have a more significant percentage of alpha-linolenic acid (56.9%–64.8%) which is the primary component of the oil. Chia seeds are gluten-free and contain biologically active antioxidant components (Muñoz et al., 2013) (Table 5.1).

Different ecosystems have substantial varying effects on quinoa (*C. quinoa* L.) and chia (*S. hispanica* L.) nutritional composition, particularly its protein and oil content, as well as its fatty acid composition. Temperature, light, soil composition, and type/variety are some of the environmental variables that have been found to impact chia seed composition (Ayerza and Coates, 2005).

PROTEIN

Quinoa has a higher protein content and quality than cereal grains while also having gluten-free and high digestibility. Quinoa has a higher total protein content than barley, oat, rice, and maize and a total protein content equal to wheat (Wright et al., 2002). Quinoa proteins are very rich in lysine, which is the limiting amino acid in most cereal grains; as compared to cereal grains in quinoa seed, there is a much higher amino acid containing higher levels of lysine (5.1%–6.4%) and methionine (0.4%–1%) (Bhargava et al., 2003). Quinoa has more histidine than barley,

TABLE 5.1
Nutritional Composition of Quinoa and Chia

Grains/Seeds (Nutrient's Amount Per 100 g)	Quinoa (*Chenopodium quinoa* L.)	Chia (*Salvia hispanica* L.)
Energy (Kcal)	367	487
Protein(g)	13.88	15.64
Fat(g)	6.06	31.84
Carbohydrates(g)	65.06	41.12
Moisture(g)	12.28	5.81
Dietary fiber (g)	7.02	33.89
Saturated fatty acid(g)	0.706	3.332
Monounsaturated fatty acid(g)	1.612	2.319
Polyunsaturated fatty acid (g)	3.289	23.655
Omega-3 (g)	0.25	17.73
Omega-6(g)	2.976	5.834

TABLE 5.2
Amino Acid Profile of Quinoa and Chia

Amino Acid (g per 100g)	Quinoa (*Chenopodium quinoa* L.)	Chia (*Salvia hispanica* L.)
Arginine	1.718	2.143
Glutamic acid	1.356	3.500
Threonine	0.818	0.709
Tryptophan	0.118	0.436
Isoleucine	0.536	0.801
Leucine	1.344	1.371
Methionine	0.181	0.588
Lysine	1.011	0.970
Cystine	0.144	0.407
Phenylalanine	0.490	1.016
Tyrosine	0.525	0.536
Histidine	0.528	0.531
Valine	0.658	0.950
Alanine	0.335	1.044
Glycine	1.037	0.943
Aspartic acid	0.594	1.689
Proline	–	0.776
Serine	0.646	1.049

Source: USDA National Nutrient Database for Standard. Reference Release 28, 2011.

soy, or wheat proteins, and its methionine and cystine level is sufficient for children (2–12 years old) and adults. The nutritional value of a food is defined by its protein quality, which is determined by the amino acid concentration, digestibility, antinutritional factors, and the ratio of tryptophan to more significant neutral amino acids (Comai et al., 2007) (Table 5.2).

The average protein content of chia seeds varies from 15% to 23%, depending on the region where the seeds were cultivated. Chia seeds have a more incredible protein content (16.54 g/100 g) than other grains such as wheat (11.8 g), rice (6.8 g), barley (11.5 g), oats (13.6 g), and corn (11.1 g) (Ayerza and Coates, 2005; Dinçoğlu and Yeşildemir, 2019). *In vitro*, the protein components of chia seed show inhibitory effects on the angiotensin-converting enzyme (ACE) (Salazar-Vega et al., 2012). The chia seed may have antihypertensive effects. Due to its low-quality protein and lack of lysine, chia seed should be eaten with lysine-rich meals when it comes to necessary amino acid content (Olivos-Lugo et al., 2010).

DIETARY FIBER

Fiber is an essential component of a balanced diet. Dietary fibers are not digested and absorbed in the small intestine; instead, they are fermented in the large intestine. Dietary fiber intake is linked to a lower risk of cardiovascular illnesses such

TABLE 5.3
Total Protein Content in Quinoa and Chia

Grains	Quinoa (*Chenopodium quinoa* L.)	Chia (*Salvia hispanica* L.)
Amount per 100 g	4.21	16.90

Source: USDA National Nutrient Database for Standard. Reference Release 28, 2011.

as stroke, vascular disease, obesity, myocardial infarction, hypertension, hyperglycemia, and hyperlipidemia. Dietary fibers are divided into two types based on their physicochemical characteristics and functions: insoluble fibers that bulk up the gut and soluble fibers that are partially or totally fermented in the colon (Lattimer and Haub, 2010; Slavin, 2013). Soluble, fermentable fibers like inulin, fructooligosaccharides, and galactooligosaccharides can cause microbial production of short-chain fatty acids (acetic, butyric, and propionic) that reduce luminal pH and promote the colonization of beneficial bacteria, so functioning as 'prebiotics' (Biesiekierski et al., 2013). Chia seeds have a total dietary fiber content of 36–40 g per 100 g, which is significantly higher than that of many grains, vegetables, and fruits such as corn, carrot, spinach, banana, pear, apple, and kiwifruit (Alfredo et al., 2009; Reyes-Caudillo et al., 2008). Dietary fiber, both insoluble and soluble, ranges from 23% to 46% and 2.5% to 7.1%, respectively. Chia seed insoluble dietary fiber can hold many times its weight in water during hydration, providing bulk and prolonging the gastrointestinal transit time. Chia contains about 5% mucilage which can also act as soluble fiber (Muñoz et al., 2012) (Table 5.3).

Quinoa seeds contain 10% total dietary fiber. Insoluble quinoa fiber, made up of galacturonic acid, arabinose, galactose, xylose, and glucose subunits, showed 78% of total quinoa fiber. Soluble quinoa fiber, mainly made up of glucose, galacturonic acid, and arabinose subunits showed 22% of total fiber (Lamothe et al., 2015).

TOTAL FATS

On average, 30.74% of lipids are found in *S. hispanica* (da Silva Marineli et al., 2014). Found that the alpha-linolenic acid (62.80 g/100 g) was the most abundant fatty acid in a study, followed by linoleic acid (18.23 g/100 g), palmitic acid (7.07 g/100 g), oleic acid (7.04 g/100 g), and stearic acid (3.36 g/100 g). Chia seeds have an average oil content of 40% of their whole weight. Hyperlipidemia, hyperglycemia, and hypertension can all be prevented and treated using omega-3 unsaturated fatty acids, that is, 60% of total oil (Capitani et al., 2012; Reyes-Caudillo et al., 2008) (Table 5.4).

The oil content in quinoa ranges from 2% to 10% (average 5–7%), which is higher than that of maize (3% to 4%) (Vega-Gálvez et al., 2010). Tang et al. (2015) reported that quinoa seed oil contains 89.4% unsaturated fatty acids and 54.2% to 58.3% PUFAs. In the total oil found in quinoa seed, on average, 50% are omega-3

TABLE 5.4
Fat Content of Chia and Quinoa

Grains (Fats g/100g)	Quinoa (*Chenopodium quinoa* L.)	Chia (*Salvia hispanica* L.)
Total Saturated fatty acids	0.706	3.33
Total monounsaturated fatty acids	1.613	2.309
Total polyunsaturated fatty acids	3.292	23.665
Omega-3 (g)	0.26	17.83
Omega-6 (g)	2.977	5.835

Source: USDA National Nutrient Database for Standard Reference Release 28, 2011.

and omega-6 fatty acids. Vitamin E and other antioxidant components of quinoa seeds protect these fatty acids from oxidation. Brain development, insulin sensitivity, cardiovascular health, prostaglandin metabolism, immunology, inflammation, and membrane function benefit from essential fatty acids (McCusker and Grant-Kels, 2010; Vega-Gálvez et al., 2010).

VITAMINS AND MINERALS

Chia seed is also found a good source of various vitamins and minerals, including niacin, zinc, calcium, phosphorus, and magnesium. Chia has a greater niacin concentration than other cereals (corn, soybeans, and rice), but its riboflavin and thiamine content is equal to corn and rice. Chia seeds provide six times the calcium, eleven times the phosphorus, and four times the potassium of 100g of milk (Muñoz et al., 2012, 2013) (Table 5.5).

TABLE 5.5
Vitamins in Grains

Grains (Vitamins mg/100g)	Quinoa (*Chenopodium quinoa* L.)	Chia (*Salvia hispanica* L.)
Vitamin A	0.39	0.55
Thiamin	0.4	0.62
Riboflavin	0.39	0.17
Niacin	1.06	8.83
Ascorbic acid	4.0–16.4	1.6
Tocopherols	3.7–6.0	0.50

Source: USDA National Nutrient Database for Standard. Reference Release 28, 2011.

TABLE 5.6
Minerals in Grain

Grains (Minerals mg/100 g)	Quinoa (*Chenopodium quinoa* L.)	Chia (*Salvia hispanica* L.)
Magnesium	0.719	335
Calcium	2.172	631
Potassium	6.938	407
Phosphorus	0.317	860
Sodium	0.370	16
Iron	255 ppm	7.72 mg
Zinc	50	4.58
Copper	13	0.9
Manganese	118	2.72

Source: USDA National Nutrient Database for Standard. Reference Release 28, 2011.

VITAMINS IN GRAINS

Quinoa seeds are high in vitamins and minerals, which are needed in the human diet to function as enzyme cofactors in metabolism, control cell growth and development, defend against oxidative damage, and improve eyesight, etc. (Fitzpatrick et al., 2012) (Table 5.6). Quinoa contains (mg/100 g) vitamin A precursor-carotene 0.39 mg, thiamin/vitamin B1 0.4 mg, riboflavin/vitamin B2 0.39 mg, niacin/vitamin B3 1.06 mg, pantothenic acid/vitamin B5 0.61 mg, pyridoxine/vitamin B6 (0.20 mg, folic acid/vitamin B9 23.5–78.1 mg, ascorbic acid/vitamin C 4.0–16.4 mg, and tocopherols/vitamin E 3.7–6.0 mg (Bhargava et al., 2003; Tang et al., 2015; Vega-Gálvez et al., 2010).

Quinoa has a total mineral (ash) than rice (0.5%), wheat (1.8%), and other cereals (3.4%). Quinoa has adequate amounts of the minerals(mg/kg) calcium 275–1487 mg, copper 2–51 mg, iron 14–168 mg, magnesium 260–5,020 mg, phosphorus 1,400–5,300 mg, potassium 75–12,000 mg, and zinc 28–48 mg to sustain a balanced human diet (Bhargava et al., 2003; Repo-Carrasco et al., 2003; Vega-Gálvez et al., 2010).

ANTIOXIDANTS

Chia seeds are rich in phenolic compounds, which have been shown in studies to have antioxidant properties. Antioxidants and phenolic compounds have been found to have health-promoting qualities and to protect against degenerative illnesses such as heart disease, cancer, diabetes, and diverticulosis (Guevara-Cruz et al., 2012). Quercetin, myricetin, kaempferol, chlorogenic acid, and 3,4 dihydroxyphenylethanol-oleanolic acid dialdehyde are all beneficial substances found in chia seeds and oil. Several *in vitro* studies have shown that these polyphenols have high antioxidant activity and that their presence is linked to reduced levels of lipid autoxidation (da Silva Marineli et al., 2014; Martínez-Cruz and Paredes-López, 2014; Reyes-Caudillo et al., 2008).

Six flavonol glycosides have been extracted from quinoa seed by Zhu et al. (2001). Seeds were shown to have antioxidant properties, indicating that they can be used as a source of antioxidants act as an excellent source of scavenging agents for free radicals. Quinoa has a tannin level of 0.051 db%, which is equivalent to amaranth, 251.5 mg/g ferulic acid, 0.8 mg/g p-coumaric acid, and 6.31 mg/g caffeic acid contents(DB) were reported (Gorinstein et al., 2008). Quinoa seeds have more antioxidant activity than other grains, according to research (rice and buckwheat).

BIOACTIVE COMPOUNDS IN QUINOA

In addition to its high nutritional value and gluten-free nature, quinoa exerts beneficial effects on high-risk group consumers, such as children, the elderly, lactose intolerant, and people with diabetes, obesity, dyslipidemia, anemia, and celiac disease. These effects have been associated with its content of protein, fiber, vitamins and minerals, fatty acids, and especially with the presence of different phytochemicals that provide quinoa a considerable advantage over other grains in terms of human nutrition and health (Navruz-Varli and Sanlier, 2016).

SAPONINS

Saponins are secondary metabolites found throughout the plant, primarily in seeds, leaves, roots, fruits, and stems. They are created to protect plants from dangerous bacteria, birds, and insects (Singh and Kaur, 2018). Saponins have sugar chains and a triterpenoid aglycone (sapogenin) in their structure and are categorized as mono-, di-, or tridesmosidic based on the number of sugar chains. Quinoa's exterior seed coat is high in saponins; thus, the content in bitter genotypes ranges from 140 to 2,300 mg/100 g dry weight, while the level in sweet genotypes ranges from 20 to 40 mg/100 g dry weight (Mastebroek et al., 2000). The main carbohydrates are glucose, arabinose, and galactose, with glucuronic acid and xylose appearing in trace amounts (Kuljanabhagavad et al., 2008). However, the majority of studies report around 20 saponins in quinoa. Yao et al. (2014) recently reported that saponin-rich quinoa seed extracts decreased nitric oxide generation and the release of proinflammatory cytokines in lipopolysaccharide-stimulated RAW 264.7 macrophages. Quinoa saponins have also been shown to inhibit 3T3-L1 adipocyte development and reduce cell viability throughout the differentiation process (Yao et al., 2015). These data suggest that quinoa saponins are capable of inhibiting adipogenesis, and therefore they appear to be natural bioactive agents efficient in adipose tissue mass regulation. Although the information on the biological actions of quinoa saponins in animals is limited, these chemicals have been shown to increase the development of humoral and cellular immune responses in mice subcutaneously vaccinated with ovalbumin (Verza et al., 2012).

PHYTOSTEROLS

Triterpenes contains a 27–30-carbon ring-based structure with hydroxyl groups present in Phytosterols (MacKay and Jones, 2011). The structure of phytosterols is similar to that of cholesterol found in animals and humans. Phytosterols compete for cholesterol's intestinal absorption and inhibit atherogenic lipoprotein synthesis in the intestines and liver, therefore lowering blood cholesterol levels (Ho and Pal, 2005).

In addition to cholesterol-lowering benefits, phytosterols have been shown to have antioxidant, anti-inflammatory, and anticancer activities. Quinoa's total phytosterol concentration ranges from 38.8 to 82.5 mg/100 g (Hernández-Ledesma, 2019), with the primary components being – sitosterol, campesterol, brassicasterol, and stigmasterol (Detmar et al., 1994). These phytosterol levels are greater than those found in barley, rye, millet, and corn (Islam et al., 2017).

PHYTOECDYSTEROIDS

Because of their structural connection with molting hormones, phytoecdysteroids are polyhydroxylated steroids that play a role in plant defense against insects. In addition to their antioxidant action, phytoecdysteroids have been shown to boost keratinocyte differentiation (Zhegn et al., 2008), increase skin thickness, and stimulate wound healing (Ehrhardt et al., 2011). Among 13 different types of phytoecdysteroids identified in quinoa, 20-hydroxyecdysone (20HE) is the most abundant, constituting 62%–90% of total quinoa phytoecdysteroids (Kumpun et al., 2011). Other minor phytoecdysteroids identified in quinoa are makisterone A, 24-epi-makisterone A, 24(28)-dehydromakisterone A, and polypodine B 24,25-dehydroinokosterone, 25,27-dehydroinokosterone, and 5b-hydroxy-24(28)-dehydromakisterone A (Kumpun et al., 2011). More recently, a 20HE-enriched quinoa extract has been found to delay/prevent the onset/occurrence of diet-induced obesity and to regulate the expression of adipocyte-specific genes in mice (Foucault et al., 2014). This anti-obesity effect might be explained by a global augment in energy expenditure, a shift in glucose metabolism toward oxidation to the detriment of lipogenesis, and a reduction in lipid absorption leading to reduced dietary lipid storage in adipose tissue (Graf et al., 2017).

HEALTH BENEFITS

Quinoa seed's high nutritional content, therapeutic qualities, and gluten-free nature may benefit a variety of consumers, including children, the elderly, high-performance athletes, lactose-intolerant consumers, osteoporosis-prone women, and people with anemia, diabetes, dyslipidemia, obesity, or celiac disease (Bhargava et al., 2003; Vega-Gálvez et al., 2010). There are limited clinical trials of quinoa seeds on animals and humans.

The intake of baby food made with quinoa (100 g twice per day for 15 days) significantly raised plasma IGF-1 levels in a childhood nutrition study among boys aged 4–5 years from respective places, but IGF-1 levels in the control group remain unchanged. IGF-1 is a hepatic peptide that stimulates growth, resulting in increased body weight and bone length. IGF-1 has been suggested as a malnutrition marker or a measure of nutritional treatment response. Quinoa seed therapy showed positive effects in the children's absorption of amino acids, as well as its excellent digestibility (95.3%), which outperformed five commercially available baby meals made from milk and soy (Ruales et al., 2002).

50 g quinoa seed (gluten-free) alternate of cereals provides a group of celiac patients for 6 weeks before and after the intervention, gastrointestinal parameters (villus height: crypt depth, surface-enterocyte cell height, and the number of intraepithelial lymphocytes per 100 enterocytes) and serum lipid levels were analyzed.

The quinoa diet improved gastrointestinal parameters, according to the research, with fewer decreases observed in total cholesterol, high-density lipoprotein (HDL), low-density lipoprotein (LDL), and triglycerides (Zevallos et al., 2014). In persons aged 18–45 years, daily intake of a quinoa cereal bar for 30 days significantly reduced triglyceride, total cholesterol, and LDL levels. Meanwhile, blood glucose levels, body weight, and blood pressure dropped (Farinazzi-Machado et al., 2012). Though the anti-diabetic benefits of quinoa have not been investigated in humans, in Wistar rats fed a high-fructose diet (31% fructose), co-administration of quinoa seeds (310 g/kg feed for five weeks) decreased substantially plasma glucose levels and oxidative stress compared to the control group (Pasko et al., 2010) (Table 5.7).

TABLE 5.7
Clinical Trials of Quinoa Seeds

Disease Treatments	Diet	Participants	Result	References
Child growth and development	Infant food formulated from quinoa (100 g×2/d for 15 days) compared with no treatment	Boys aged 50–65 months from low-income families	Increase Plasma levels of IGF-1, a marker of malnutrition, which help in increasing body weight	(Ruales et al., 2002)
Celiac disease	Cooked quinoa (50 g/d for 6 weeks)	19 celiac patients	All gastrointestinal parameters (villus height: crypt depth), surface-enterocyte cell height, number of intra-epithelial lymphocytes per 100 enterocytes) improved following quinoa diet; serum lipid levels remained regular with a slight decrease in total cholesterol, LDL, HDL, and triglycerides	(Zevallos et al., 2014)
Risk of cardiovascular disease	Quinoa cereal bar daily for 30 days	22 students aged 18–45 years	Lower triglycerides, cholesterol and LDL	(Farinazzi-Machado et al., 2012)
Postmenopausal symptoms	Quinoa flakes (QF) compared with corn flakes (CF), 25 g/d for 4 weeks	35 postmenopausal women with excess weight	Increased protein and fiber intake but no effect on total caloric intake. lower triglycerides, TBARS cholesterol, LDL, and increase glutathione	(De Carvalho et al., 2014)

LDL: low-density lipoprotein, HDL: high-density lipoprotein, TBARS: Thiobarbituric acid-reactive substances.

TABLE 5.8
Clinical Trial of Chia Seeds

Disease Treatments	Diet	Participants	Result	References
Type-2 diabetes	15 g/1000 kcal chia seed 12 weeks	Aged 18–75 Type 2 DM 11 male, 9 female	Decrease in systolic blood pressure, hs-CRP, HbA1C, and von Willebrand factor – Increased plasma ALA and EPA levels	(Vuksan et al., 2007)
Overweight adults	25 g whole chia seed or placebo flour two times per day 12 weeks	Aged 20–70 healthy overweight/ obese 28 male, 48 female	No effect on body composition, inflammation, oxidative stress, blood pressure, and lipoproteins. Increase in plasma ALA levels, no change in EPA, DHA levels	(Nieman et al., 2009)
Postmenopausal symptoms	25 g milled chia seed 7 weeks	25 g milled chia seed	Increase in ALA and EPA levels, no effect on DHA levels	(Jin et al., 2012)
Health purpose	0, 7, 15, or 25 g whole or milled chia seed in 50 g bread. Postprandial (15., 30., 45., 60., 90., 120. min)	13 healthy individuals	Decrease in blood glucose levels in a dose-dependent manner whether it is milled or whole chia	(H. Ho et al., 2013)

ALA: α-linolenic acid, EPA: Eicosapentaenoic acid, DHA: Docosahexaenoic acid.

Chia seeds have many health benefits; because of their high omega-3 fatty acid content, daily use of chia seeds may enhance plasma omega-3 fraction levels (Jin et al., 2012; Vuksan et al., 2007) (Table 5.8). However, although *in vitro* and animal research show that it lowers blood pressure, human trials show mixed outcomes. Furthermore, chia seed intake may support the reduction of high-sensitivity C-reactive protein levels (Jin et al., 2012; Toscano et al., 2014; Vuksan et al., 2007).

On ten healthy postmenopausal women, the effects of consuming 25 g milled chia seeds for seven weeks were studied. Intake of chia seeds increased plasma levels of eicosapentaenoic acid (EPA) and alpha-linolenic acid (ALA) by 30% and 138%, respectively (Jin et al., 2012). Higher dietary intake of omega-3 fatty acids from both marine (EPA and DHA) and plant sources (ALA) is helpful to a lower risk of death from cardiovascular diseases (Koh et al., 2015). According to (Vuksan et al., 2007), people with type 2 diabetes on medication were given 37 grams of chia seeds daily (added in white bread). The high fiber content of chia seed helped manage hyperglycemia and lower systolic blood pressure. Peoples with over body weight divided into two groups was given them 4 g chia seeds, oats, palm, and soy powder dissolved in 250 mL water twice daily for two months, along with specific calorie changes in the regular diet. In comparison to the control group, the experimental group's body weight, waist circumference, and basal metabolic rate all decreased significantly. Insulin resistance, lipid levels, and C-reactive protein levels all decreased significantly. On the other hand, total cholesterol, blood sugar, and total plasma insulin levels had no significant change (Guevara-Cruz et al., 2012).

BIBLIOGRAPHY

Alfredo, V.-O., Gabriel, R.-R., Luis, C.-G., and David, B.-A. (2009). Physicochemical properties of a fibrous fraction from chia (Salvia hispanica L.). *LWT-Food Sci Technol* 42(1):168–173.

Ayerza, R. and Coates, W. (2005). *Chia: Rediscovering a Forgotten Crop of the Aztecs.* University of Arizona Press.

Bhargava, A., Shukla, S., and Ohri, D. (2003). Genetic variability and heritability of selected traits during different cuttings of vegetable Chenopodium. *Indian J Genet Plant Breed* 63(4):359–360.

Biesiekierski, J. R., Muir, J. G., and Gibson, P. R. (2013). Is gluten a cause of gastrointestinal symptoms in people without celiac disease? *Current Allergy Asthma Rep* 13(6):631–638.

Capitani, M. I., Spotorno, V., Nolasco, S. M., and Tomás, M. C. (2012). Physicochemical and functional characterization of by-products from chia (Salvia hispanica L.) seeds of Argentina. *LWT-Food Sci Technol* 45(1):94–102.

Chauhan, G. S., Eskin, N. A. M., and Tkachuk, R. (1992). Nutrients and antinutrients in quinoa seed. *Cereal Chem* 69(1):85–88.

Chludil, H. D., Corbino, G. B., and Leicach, S. R. (2008). Soil quality effects on Chenopodium album flavonoid content and antioxidant potential. *J Agri Food Chem* 56(13):5050–5056.

Comai, S., Bertazzo, A., Bailoni, L., Zancato, M., Costa, C. V. L., and Allegri, G. (2007). The content of protein and non proteic (free and protein-bound) tryptophan in quinoa and cereal flours. *Food Chem* 100(4):1350–1355.

Coorey, R., Grant, A., and Jayasena, V. (2012). Effect of chia flour incorporation on the nutritive quality and consumer acceptance of chips. *J Food Res* 1:85–95.

da Silva Marineli, R., Moraes, É. A., Lenquiste, S. A., Godoy, A. T., Eberlin, M. N., and Maróstica Jr, M. R. (2014). Chemical characterization and antioxidant potential of Chilean chia seeds and oil (Salvia hispanica L.). *LWT-Food Sci Technol* 59(2):1304–1310.

De Carvalho, F. G., Ovídio, P. P., Padovan, G. J., Jordao Junior, A. A., Marchini, J. S., and Navarro, A. M. (2014). Metabolic parameters of postmenopausal women after quinoa or corn flakes intake–a prospective and double-blind study. *Int J Food Sci Nutr* 65(3):380–385.

Detmar, M., Dumas, M., Bonte, F., Meybeck, A., and Orfanos, C. E. (1994). Effects of ecdysterone on the differentiation of normal human keratinocytes in-vitro. *Eur J Dermatol* 4(7):558–562.

Dinçoğlu, A. H., and Yeşildemir, Ö. (2019). A renewable source as functional foodhia seed. *Current Nutr Food Sci* 15(4):327–337.

Ehrhardt, C., Wessels, J. T., Wuttke, W., and Seidlová-Wuttke, D. (2011). The effects of 20-hydroxyecdysone and 17β-estradiol on the skin of ovariectomized rats. *Menopause* 18(3):323–327.

Farinazzi-Machado, F. M. V., Barbalho, S. M., Oshiiwa, M., Goulart, R., and Pessan Junior, O. (2012). Use of cereal bars with quinoa (Chenopodium quinoa W.) to reduce risk factors related to cardiovascular diseases. *Food Sci Technol* 32:239–244.

Fitzpatrick, T. B., Basset, G. J. C., Borel, P., Carrari, F., DellaPenna, D., Fraser, P. D., Hellmann, H., Osorio, S., Rothan, C., and Valpuesta, V. (2012). Vitamin deficiencies in humans: can plant science help? *The Plant Cell* 24(2):395–414.

Foucault, A.-S., Even, P., Lafont, R., Dioh, W., Veillet, S., Tomé, D., Huneau, J.-F., Hermier, D., and Quignard-Boulangé, A. (2014). Quinoa extract enriched in 20-hydroxyecdysone affects energy homeostasis and intestinal fat absorption in mice fed a high-fat diet. *Physiol Behav* 128:226–231.

Giaretta, D., Lima, V. A., and Carpes, S. T. (2018). Improvement of fatty acid profile in loaves of bread supplemented with Kinako flour and chia seed. *Innov Food Sci Emerg Technol* 49:211–214.

Gorinstein, S., Lojek, A., Číž, M., Pawelzik, E., Delgado-Licon, E., Medina, O. J., Moreno, M., Salas, I. A., and Goshev, I. (2008). Comparison of composition and antioxidant capacity of some cereals and pseudocereals. *Int J Food Sci Technol* 43(4):629–637.

Graf, B. L., Kamat, S., Cheong, K. Y., Komarnytsky, S., Driscoll, M., and Di, R. (2017). Phytoecdysteroid-enriched quinoa seed leachate enhances healthspan and mitochondrial metabolism in Caenorhabditiselegans. *J Functional Foods* 37:1–7.

Guevara-Cruz, M., Tovar, A. R., Aguilar-Salinas, C. A., Medina-Vera, I., Gil-Zenteno, L., Hernández-Viveros, I., López-Romero, P., Ordaz-Nava, G., Canizales-Quinteros, S., and Guillen Pineda, L. E. (2012). A dietary pattern including nopal, chia seed, soy protein, and oat reduces serum triglycerides and glucose intolerance in patients with metabolic syndrome. *J Nutr* 142(1):64–69.

GuhaBakshi, D. N., Sensarma, P., and Pal, D. C. (1999). *Lexicon of Medicinal Plants in India.* Naya Prokash.

Hernández-Ledesma, B. (2019). Quinoa (Chenopodium quinoa Willd.) as a source of bioactive compounds: A review. *Bioactive Compounds Health Dis* 2(3):27–47.

Ho, H., Lee, A. S., Jovanovski, E., Jenkins, A. L., Desouza, R., and Vuksan, V. (2013). Effect of whole and ground Salba seeds (Salvia Hispanica L.) on postprandial glycemia in healthy volunteers: A randomized controlled, dose-response trial. *Eur J Clin Nutr* 67(7):786–788.

Ho, S. S. and Pal, S. (2005). Margarine phytosterols decrease the secretion of atherogenic lipoproteins from HepG2 liver and Caco2 intestinal cells. *Atherosclerosis* 182(1):29–36.

Islam, M. A., Jeong, B.-G., Jung, J., Shin, E.-C., Choi, S.-G., and Chun, J. (2017). Phytosterol determination and method validation for selected nuts and seeds. *Food Anal Methods* 10(10):3225–3234.

James, L. E. A. (2009). Quinoa (Chenopodium quinoa Willd.): Composition, chemistry, nutritional, and functional properties. *Adv Food Nutr Res* 58:1–31.

Jin, F., Nieman, D. C., Sha, W., Xie, G., Qiu, Y., and Jia, W. (2012). Supplementation of milled chia seeds increases plasma ALA and EPA in postmenopausal women. *Plant Foods Human Nutr* 67(2):105–110.

Koh, A. S., Pan, A., Wang, R., Odegaard, A. O., Pereira, M. A., Yuan, J.-M., and Koh, W.-P. (2015). The association between dietary omega-3 fatty acids and cardiovascular death: the Singapore Chinese Health Study. *Eur J Prevent Cardiol* 22(3):364–372.

Koziol, M. J. (1993). *Quinoa: A Potential New Oil Crop. New Crops.* J. Janick and J. E. Simon (Eds.), Wiley, New York, 328–336.

Kuljanabhagavad, T., Thongphasuk, P., Chamulitrat, W., and Wink, M. (2008). Triterpene saponins from Chenopodium quinoa Willd. *Phytochemistry* 69(9):1919–1926.

Kumpun, S., Maria, A., Crouzet, S., Evrard-Todeschi, N., Girault, J.-P., and Lafont, R. (2011). Ecdysteroids from Chenopodium quinoa Willd., an ancient Andean crop of high nutritional value. *Food Chem* 125(4):1226–1234.

Lamothe, L. M., Srichuwong, S., Reuhs, B. L., and Hamaker, B. R. (2015). Quinoa (Chenopodium quinoa W.) and amaranth (Amaranthuscaudatus L.) provide dietary fibers high in pectic substances and xyloglucans. *Food Chem* 167:490–496.

Lattimer, J. M. and Haub, M. D. (2010). Effects of dietary fiber and its components on metabolic health. *Nutrients* 2(12):1266–1289.

MacKay, D. S. and Jones, P. J. H. (2011). Phytosterols in human nutrition: Type, formulation, delivery, and physiological function. *Eur J Lipid Sci Technol* 113(12):1427–1432.
Martínez-Cruz, O. and Paredes-López, O. (2014). Phytochemical profile and nutraceutical potential of chia seeds (Salvia hispanica L.) by ultra-high-performance liquid chromatography. *J Chromatogr A* 1346:43–48.
Mastebroek, H. D., Limburg, H., Gilles, T., and Marvin, H. J. P. (2000). Occurrence of sapogenins in leaves and seeds of quinoa (Chenopodium quinoa Willd). *J Sci Food Agri* 80(1):152–156.
McCusker, M. M., and Grant-Kels, J. M. (2010). Healing fats of the skin: The structural and immunologic roles of the ω-6 and ω-3 fatty acids. *Clinics Dermat* 28(4):440–451.
Muñoz, L. A., Cobos, A., Diaz, O., and Aguilera, J. M. (2012). Chia seeds: Microstructure, mucilage extraction, and hydration. *J Food Eng* 108(1):216–224.
Muñoz, L. A., Cobos, A., Diaz, O., and Aguilera, J. M. (2013). Chia seed (Salvia hispanica): An ancient grain and a new functional food. *Food Rev Int* 29(4):394–408.
Navruz-Varli, S. and Sanlier, N. (2016). Nutritional and health benefits of quinoa (Chenopodium quinoa Willd.). *J Cereal Sci* 69:371–376.
Nieman, D. C., Cayea, E. J., Austin, M. D., Henson, D. A., McAnulty, S. R., and Jin, F. (2009). Chia seed does not promote weight loss or alter disease risk factors in overweight adults. *Nutr Res* 29(6):414–418.
Olivos-Lugo, B. L., Valdivia-López, M. Á., and Tecante, A. (2010). Thermal and physicochemical properties and nutritional value of the protein fraction of Mexican chia seed (Salvia hispanica L.). *Food Sci Techno Int* 16(1):89–96.
Oshodi, A. A., Ogungbenle, H. N., and Oladimeji, M. O. (1999). Chemical composition, nutritionally valuable minerals, and functional properties of benniseed (Sesamum radiatum), pearl millet (Pennisetum typhoides), and quinoa (Chenopodium quinoa) flours. *Int J Food Sci Nutr* 50(5):325–331.
Pasko, P., Barton, H., Zagrodzki, P., Izewska, A., Krosniak, M., Gawlik, M., Gawlik, M., and Gorinstein, S. (2010). Effect of diet supplemented with quinoa seeds on oxidative status in plasma and selected tissues of high fructose-fed rats. *Plant Foods Human Nutr* 65(2):146–151.
Prakash, D. and Pal, M. (1998). Chenopodium: Seed protein, fractionation, and amino acid composition. *Int J Food Sci Nutr* 49(4):271–275.
Rendón-Villalobos, J. R., Ortíz-Sánchez, A., and Flores-Huicochea, E. (2018). Nutritionally enhanced foods incorporating Chía seed. In *Therapeutic Foods*. Elsevier, 257–281.
Repo-Carrasco, R., Espinoza, C., and Jacobsen, S.-E. (2003). Nutritional value and use of the Andean crops quinoa (Chenopodium quinoa) and kañiwa (Chenopodium pallidicaule). *Food Rev Int* 19(1–2):179–189.
Reyes-Caudillo, E., Tecante, A., and Valdivia-López, M. A. (2008). Dietary fibre content and antioxidant activity of phenolic compounds present in Mexican chia (Salvia hispanica L.) seeds. *Food Chem* 107(2):656–663.
Ruales, J., Grijalva, Y. de, Lopez-Jaramillo, P., and Nair, B. M. (2002). The nutritional quality of an infant food from quinoa and its effect on the plasma level of insulin-like growth factor-1 (IGF-1) in undernourished children. *Int J Food Sci Nutr* 53(2):143–154.
Salazar-Vega, I. M., Segura-Campos, M. R., Chel-Guerrero, L. A., and Betancur-Ancona, D. A. (2012). Antihypertensive and antioxidant effects of functional foods containing chia (Salvia hispanica) protein hydrolysates. In: *Scientific, Health and Social Aspects of the Food Industry*. B. Valdez (Ed.). InTech, Croatia.
Singh, B. and Kaur, A. (2018). Control of insect pests in crop plants and stored food grains using plant saponins: A review. *Lwt* 87:93–101.
Slavin, J. (2013). Fiber and prebiotics: Mechanisms and health benefits. *Nutrients* 5(4):1417–1435.

Tang, Y., Li, X., Chen, P. X., Zhang, B., Hernandez, M., Zhang, H., Marcone, M. F., Liu, R., and Tsao, R. (2015). Characterization of fatty acid, carotenoid, tocopherol/tocotrienol compositions, and antioxidant activities in seeds of three Chenopodium quinoa Willd. Genotypes. *Food Chem* 174:502–508.

Toscano, L. T., da Silva, C. S. O., Toscano, L. T., de Almeida, A. E. M., da Cruz Santos, A., and Silva, A. S. (2014). Chia flour supplementation reduces blood pressure in hypertensive subjects. *Plant Foods Human Nutr* 69(4):392–398.

Vega-Gálvez, A., Miranda, M., Vergara, J., Uribe, E., Puente, L., and Martínez, E. A. (2010). Nutrition facts and functional potential of quinoa (Chenopodium quinoa willd.), an ancient Andean grain: A review. *J Sci Food Agri* 90(15):2541–2547.

Verza, S. G., Silveira, F., Cibulski, S., Kaiser, S., Ferreira, F., Gosmann, G., Roehe, P. M., and Ortega, G. G. (2012). Immunoadjuvant activity, toxicity assays, and determination by UPLC/Q-TOF-MS of triterpenic saponins from Chenopodium quinoa seeds. *J Agri Food Chem* 60(12):3113–3118.

Vuksan, V., Whitham, D., Sievenpiper, J. L., Jenkins, A. L., Rogovik, A. L., Bazinet, R. P., Vidgen, E., and Hanna, A. (2007). Supplementation of conventional therapy with the novel grain Salba (*Salvia hispanica* L.) improves major and emerging cardiovascular risk factors in type 2 diabetes: Results of a randomized controlled trial. *Diabetes Care* 30(11):2804–2810.

Wright, K. H., Pike, O. A., Fairbanks, D. J., and Huber, C. S. (2002). Composition of Atriplexhortensis, sweet and bitter Chenopodium quinoa seeds. *J Food Sci* 67(4):1383–1385.

Yao, Y., Yang, X., Shi, Z., and Ren, G. (2014). Anti-inflammatory activity of saponins from quinoa (Chenopodium quinoa Willd.) seeds in lipopolysaccharide-stimulated RAW 264.7 macrophages cells. *Journal Food Sci* 79(5):H1018–H1023.

Yao, Y., Zhu, Y., Gao, Y., Shi, Z., Hu, Y., and Ren, G. (2015). Suppressive effects of saponin-enriched extracts from quinoa on 3T3-L1 adipocyte differentiation. *Food Function* 6(10):3282–3290.

Zevallos, V. F., Herencia, I. L., Chang, F., Donnelly, S., Ellis, J. H., and Ciclitira, P. J. (2014). Gastrointestinal effects of eating quinoa (Chenopodium quinoa Willd.) in celiac patients. *Official J Am College Gastroenterol| ACG* 109(2):270–278.

Zhegn, G. Y., Wu, X., Li, Y. L., Zhang, J. H., and Wang, W. J. (2008). Preparation and dose-effect analysis of ecdysterone cream for promoting wound healing. *J Southern Medical University* 28(5):828–831.

Zhu, N., Sheng, S., Li, D., Lavoie, E. J., Karwe, M. V., Rosen, R. T., and Ho, C. (2001). Antioxidative flavonoid glycosides from quinoa seeds (Chenopodium quinoa Willd). *J Food Lipids* 8(1):37–44.

6 Quinoa and Chia – Types, Composition, and Therapeutic Properties

We have discussed in earlier chapters that quinoa (*Chenopodium quinoa* Willd.) is a dicotyledonous crop and grown in the Andean region, including Colombia, Peru, Ecuador, Argentina, Chile, and Bolivia (Ruiz et al., 2014; Fuentes et al., 2012). Quinoa has a higher nutritional value than many traditional grains, even if cultivated up to 4,500 m a.s.l. (Tapia, 1997). For instance, Amarilla de Marangoni and Blanca de Junın, two commercial varieties, have grown significantly in the Andes of southern Peru (Ormachea and Quispe, 1993). Most varieties of quinoa commonly differ in the morphology, phenology, and chemical composition of the tissues (Bertero et al., 2004). The quinoa (a dicot plant) is not an actual grain, like typical cereal (monocot) grains; it is instead a fruit, so that it has been called a pseudo-cereal and even a pseudo-oilseed. It is also because of its unusual composition and exceptional balance between oil, protein, and fat (Cusack, 1984). Its high protein content is the exceptional nutritious component of interest regarding essential amino acids. Quinoa seeds are also rich sources of essential (poly-) unsaturated fatty acids, minerals, and a sizeable antioxidant capacity (Vega-Gálvez, 2010; Abugoch James, 2009; Paśko et al., 2009). Quinoa is gluten-free, so suitable for celiac patients (Peñas et al., 2014). To meet the increasing demand for raw quinoa seeds, the countries like Bolivia and Peru expanded the agricultural production area for the crop. It was accompanied by unsustainability, resulting in the depletion of natural vegetation. Growing quinoa on contaminated soils brought severe consequences to the indigenous population (Bazile et al., 2016; Perreault, 2013; Jacobsen, 2011; Biodiversity International, 2007).

Quinoa seeds are round and flattened, having a diameter from about 1.5 to 4 mm; about 350 seeds weigh 1 g (Ruales and Nair, 1993). Seed size and color are variable (Mujica, 1994). The color and tint of the seeds vary from white to grey and black. Some varieties potentially have tones of yellow, rose, red and purple, and violet, often with very colorful mixes in the same panicle, where black is dominant over red and yellow, which are dominant to white seed color. The quinoa seeds were first classified based on the color of the plant and fruits. Later it was done based on the morphological types of the plant. Despite the wide variation observed, quinoa has considered one single species (Valencia-Chamorro, 2003).

DOI: 10.1201/9781003080770-6

Quinoa content is rich in minerals such as calcium, iron, zinc, magnesium, and manganese, which give the grains high value for different target populations: for instance, adults and children benefit from calcium for bones and iron for blood functions (Kozioł, 1992; Repo-Carrasco et al., 2003). Antioxidant properties conferred by vitamin E and ω-3 fatty acids, plus the neuronal activity of tryptophan amino acid and vitamin B complex, can be powerful aids in brain function. Besides, zinc helps the immunological system, and magnesium is also essential during neuromessengers and neuron modulators. Quinoa also improves some insulin-like forms, active as growth hormones (Ruales et al., 2002). The low glycemic index makes quinoa suitable for diabetic patients (low fructose and glucose), as Oshodi et al. (1999) mentioned. Celiac and lactose-intolerant subjects should also be quinoa consumers because of their gluten-free nature and their rich protein levels, similar to milk casein quality (Herencia et al., 1999).

GENERAL FEATURES

Quinoa seeds correspond to the campylotropous type of Boesewinkel and Bouman (1984), i.e., the embryo is peripheral, and a basal body (cf. Bouman, 1984) is present in the seeds as a storage tissue or perisperm (Figure 6.1). In the mature seed, the endosperm is present only in the micropylar region of the seed. It consists of one to two cell-layered tissue surrounding the hypocotyl-radicle axis of the embryo (Figures 6.2 and 6.3). A rectilinear vascular strand runs throughout the funiculus (Figures 6.1 and 6.2). Quinoa seeds are disseminated with the pericarp covering the seed (Figures 6.1–6.4). The pericarp was two layered (Figure 6.4). The cells of the outer layer were large and papillose in shape. The inner layer was discontinuous, and its cells were tangentially stretched. The seed coat consisted of two layers of cells (Figures 6.3, 6.4, and 6.7): the exotesta and the endotegmen. The cells of the exotesta were large with very thick walls and reduced cytoplasm; starch grains and crystals (Figure 6.7) were occasionally

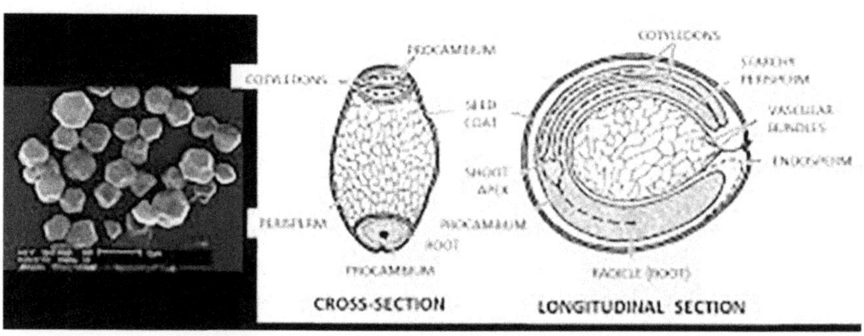

FIGURE 6.1 Quinoa seed.

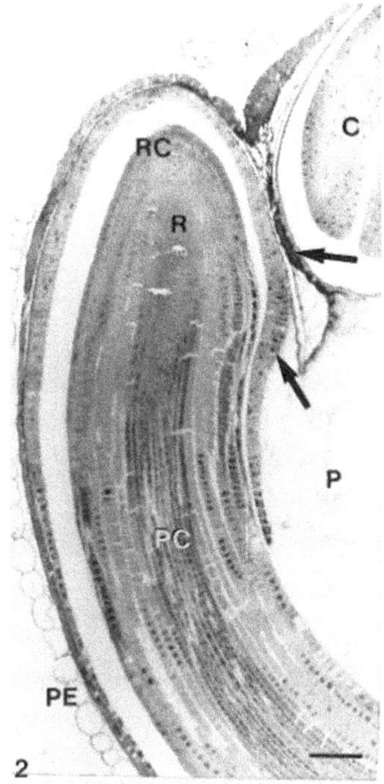

FIGURE 6.2 A section of part of the hypocotyl-radicle axis: C, Cotyledon; P, perisperm; PE, pericarp; R, radicle tip; RC, root cap; endosperm (black arrow). Bar¯100 lm.

observed in the cytoplasm of these cells. The cells of the endotegmen showed small thickenings in the inner walls (Figure 6.7). The endotesta and the exotegmen were collapsed, persisting only as cell walls.

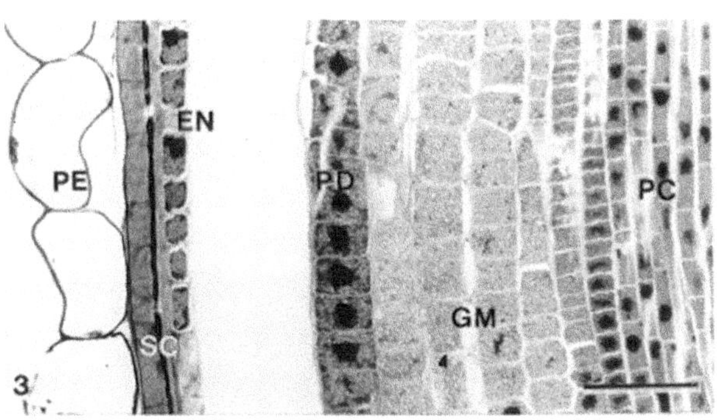

FIGURE 6.3 Enlargement of Fig. 2. EN, endosperm; GM, ground meristem; PC, procambium; P.D., protoderm; PE, pericarp; SC, seed coat. Bar¯50 lm.

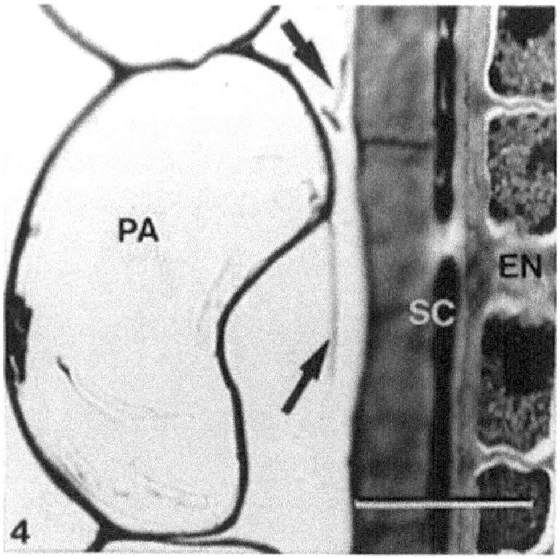

FIGURE 6.4 Detail of pericarp and seed coat. The outer layer of the pericarp with papillose cells (P.A.) and the inner discontinuous layer with tangentially stretched cells (black arrows) are shown. One-layered seed coat (SC) in contact with the endosperm (EN). Bar¯25 lm.

PERISPERM

The perisperm consisted of uniform, nonliving, thin-walled cells. The cells were full of starch grains which were angular in shape (Figure 6.5); nuclei and other cytoplasmic organelles were absent at this stage. Simple and compound starch grains occurred in the same cells (Figure 6.6). Cell walls and starch grains stained with the PAS reaction; starch grains also stained with iodine-potassium iodide. The single grains varied in diameter from approx. 0±5 to 1±0 µm. Compound structures, consisting of oblong aggregates of simple grains, were around 20–25 µm in size. The endosperm, The endosperm of the mature seed, consisted only of a one–two cell layer in the micropylar region, enveloping the hypocotyl-radicle axis. Endosperm cells had thick rigid outer-cell walls. Cell walls stained with the

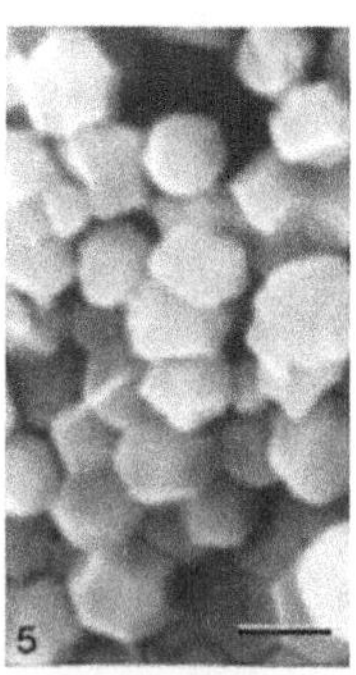

FIGURE 6.5 Scanning electron micrograph of a perisperm cell showing single starch grains. Bar¯1 lm.

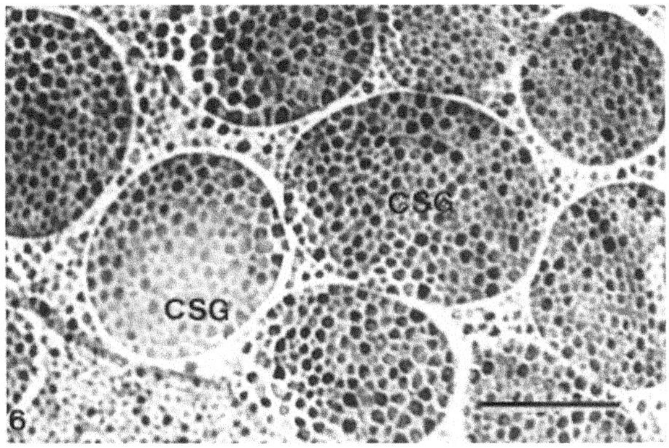

FIGURE 6.6 Light microscopy of a perisperm cell section shows single and compound starch grains (CSG). The section is stained with PAS. Bar¯10 lm.

PAS reaction and Toluidine blue O. The cuticle, representing the nucellar cuticle, is stained with Sudan black B. The cells have living cytoplasm with round or lobed nuclei. The proportion of normal constituents, i.e., cytoplasm, endoplasmic reticulum, proplastids, and mitochondria, was tiny. Endoplasmic reticulum occurred as closely packed sheets of cisternae. Proplastids were recognized by the presence of deposits of phytoferritin (cf. Robards and Humpherson, 1967). Protein and lipid bodies occupied most of the cytoplasm. Lipids were determined by cytochemical staining with Sudan black B. Endosperm protein bodies varied in diameter from 1 to 3 μm and consisted of a proteinaceous matrix containing one or more globoid crystals.

The globoid crystals stained meta chromatically with Toluidine blue O and the proteinaceous region of the protein bodies stained with bromophenol blue, Coomassie brilliant blue, Fast green FCF, and acid fuchsin. As explained in the figures, EDX analysis from powdered preparations revealed that globoid crystals contained P, K, and Mg. Embryo The embryo consisted of a hypocotyl-radicle axis and two cotyledons; in the axis, the meristem of the root with the root cap (Figures 6.1–6.10) and the apical meristem of the shoot were distinguishable. Protoderm, procambium palisade, and spongy tissues were visible in the cotyledons and protoderm. Procambium and ground meristem were visible in the axis (Figures 6.1–6.10). All the embryo cells had thin primary cell walls stained with PAS, Fast green FCF, acid fuchsin, and Toluidine blue O. Nuclei were round or lobed and occupied the cell center. The endoplasmic reticulum was present in the form of closely packed sheets of cisternae (Figures 6.1–6.10). Proplastids occurred in the protoderm and mesophyll of the cotyledons and the ground meristem of the axis; they contained clusters of dense particles of phytoferritin and, occasionally, starch grains (Figures 6.1–6.10).

Vacuole-like structures were seen in proplastids (Figures 6.1–6.10). Embryo cells of the apical meristem stored abundant protein and lipids in the form of protein and lipid bodies (Figures 6.1–6.8). The presence of lipids was determined by staining with Sudan black B. Protein in the protein bodies was determined by staining

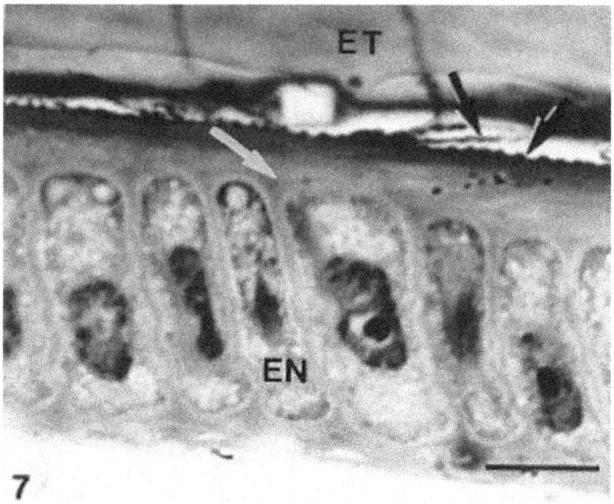

FIGURE 6.7 Light microscopy of a section of the micropylar endosperm (EN). Endosperm cells have thick outer cell walls (white arrow)—cells of the exotesta (ET) with a crystal. Cells of the endotegmen showed thickenings in their inner walls (black arrows). The section is stained with PAS and Toluidine blue O. Bar¯10 lm.

with bromophenol blue, Coomassie brilliant blue, acid fuchsin, and Fast green FCF. Protein bodies contained one or more globoid crystals in the proteinaceous matrix (Figures 6.1–6.4) and varied in diameter from 0±5 to 3 μm. Procambium and apical meristems contained small protein bodies. The proteinaceous matrix was less electron-dense in the protein bodies of the protoderm and frequently also in the smaller protein bodies of the other tissues. They stained metachromatically with Toluidine blue O (Figures 6.3–6.8). EDX analysis of globoid crystals from powdered preparation of different embryo tissues revealed that they contained P, K, and Mg. For the three elements, values were not significantly different between cotyledons and the axis. Traces of other minerals were not detected.

GENETIC DIVERSITY AND VARIETIES

The Andean Region is among one of the eight centers of crop origin and diversity. The most remarkable genetic diversity of wild and cultivated quinoa is found in the Andean farmer's fields. Quinoa has received the most dedication and support among Andean crops in Ecuador, Peru, and Bolivia. Assessments of the available genetic variability have allowed quinoas to be categorized into five major groups based on their adaptations and some highly heritable morphological traits, which are easily detectable and managed in the whole distribution area.

The primary five groups of quinoas, according to Lescano (1989) and Tapia (1990), are:

1. Sea-level quinoas: Found in Linares and Concepci6n (Chile) areas at 36° South latitude. These sea-level quinoa plants are more or less robust plants, 1.0–1.4 m tall, branched growth, and produce refined cream-colored

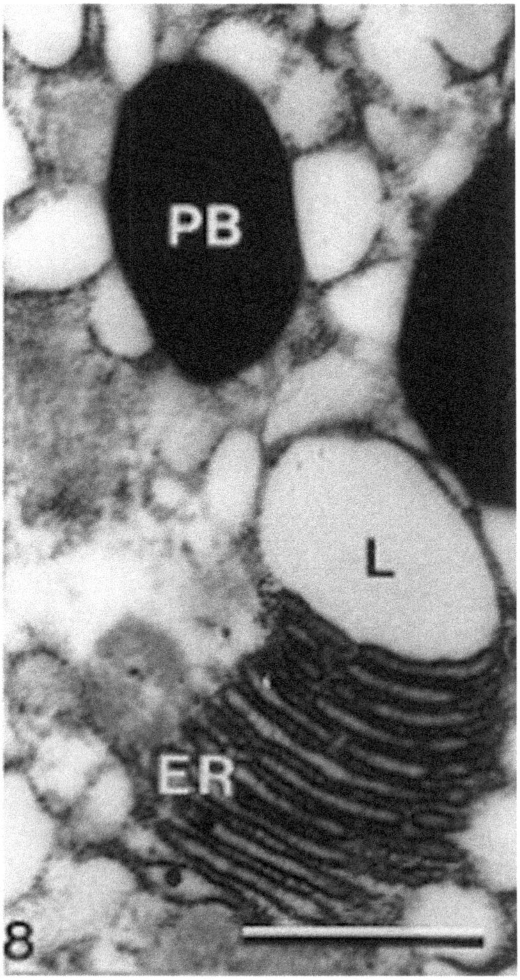

FIGURE 6.8 Section of part of a cell showing endoplasmic reticulum (ER) forming closely packed sheets of cisternae. Bar¯1 lm.

Figures 6.8–6.12 Transmission electron micrographs of sections of the endosperm. Tissues were fixed with glutaraldehyde and stained with uranyl acetate and lead citrate. Empty areas in Figures 6.11 and 6.12 contained globoid crystals before they were chipped out during sectioning.

grains (Chullpi type). These quinoas have remarkable similarities with Chenopodium nuttalliae (Huahzontle) and are only grown in the Mexico region at 20° North Latitude.

2. Valley quinoas: These adapt between 2,500 and 3,500 m. Valley quinoas were characterized by their height of up to 2.5 m or more, are extensively branching with lax inflorescences, and are usually resistant to mildew (*Peronospora farinosa*).

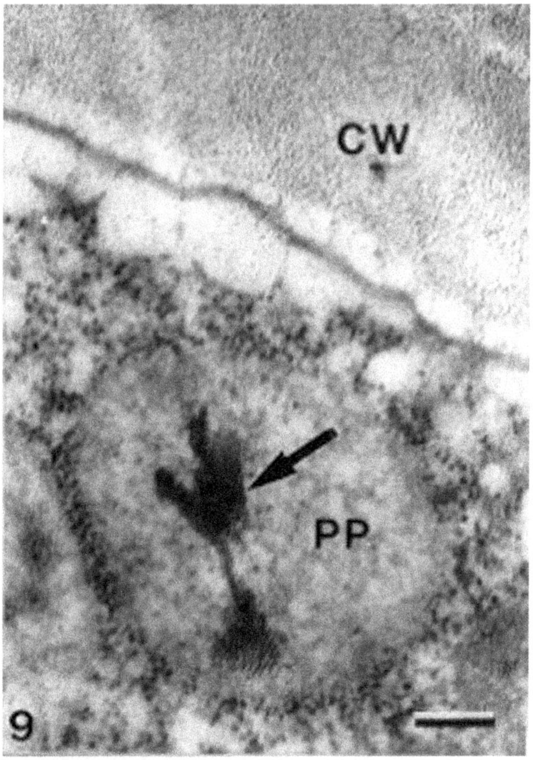

FIGURE 6.9 Proplastid (PP) of a cell of the endosperm with clusters of electron-dense particles of phytoferritin (black arrow); CW, cell wall. Bar¯1 lm.

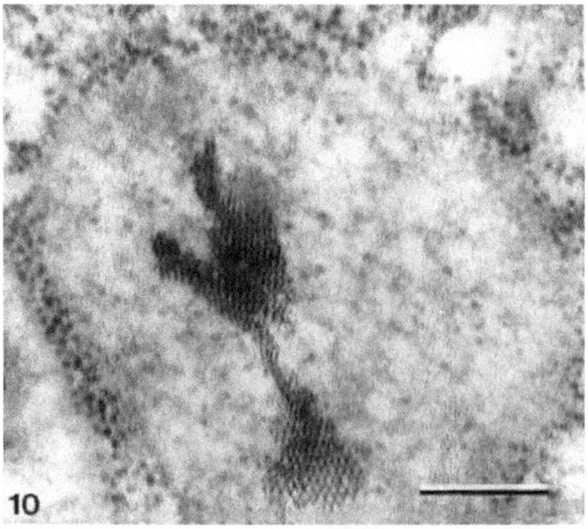

FIGURE 6.10 Enlargement of Figure 6.10. Bar¯1 lm.

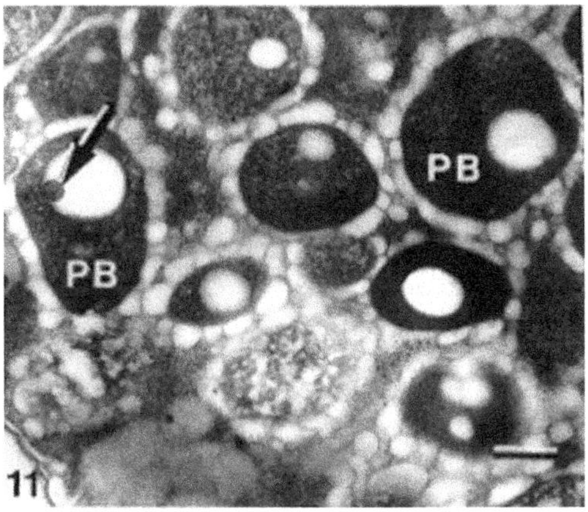

FIGURE 6.11 Section of an endosperm cell showing protein bodies (PB); a black arrow indicates a globoid crystal. Bar¯1 lm.

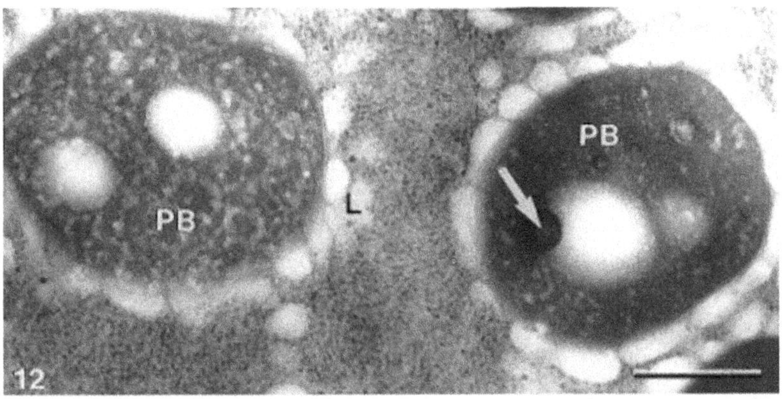

FIGURE 6.12 An enlargement section of a cell of the endosperm showing lipid bodies (L) and two protein bodies (PB), one of them with a globoid crystal (white arrow). Bar¯1 lm.

3. Altiplano quinoas: They develop in more extensive regions between 3,600 and 3,800 masl in the area of the Peruvian-Bolivian Altiplano. The grains with the most specialized uses and variability of characters are produced. The height of the plants grows to 0.5–1.5 m, with a stem ending in a generally compact main panicle. This group contains many improved varieties susceptible to mildew when taken to humid/wet areas.
4. Salt flat quinoas: These quinoa seeds grow in the driest and flat salt areas to the south of the Bolivian Altiplano having about 300 mm of precipitation. Here they are grown as a single crop with 1 m × 1m in holes to use the little humidity available efficiently. This quinoa has the largest grain size (>2.2 mm in diameter) and is known as 'Royal Quinoa'. The grains of royal quinoa are characterized by very thick pericarp and significant content of saponin.

5. Quinoas of the Yungas: A group of quinoas shows branched development and adapted to the climatic conditions of the Bolivian Yungas at altitudes between 1,500 and 2,000 masl. They are green plants with a height up to 2.20 m and take orange color when in bloom. According to Mujica (1992), quinoas have high genetic diversity and show variability in the plant color, inflorescence, and seed, which confers them with adaptability to different ecological conditions (soil, rainfall, temperature, altitude, resistance to frost, drought, salinity or acidity).

Among all the main varieties known in the Andean Region, 22 varieties are obtained by genetic improvement through hybridization and selection in Bolivia. Many bitter varieties known as 'Royal Quinoa' which includes several local races: Royal white, Mañiqueña, Huallata, Toledo, Pink Mok'o, Tres Hermanos, K'ellu, Orange Canchis, Pisankalla, Pink Pandela, Perlasa, Achachino, Hilo, White rose, Mok'o, Timsa, Lipeña, Chillpi Amapola, Pink Chillpi, Utusaya, and Pink Canchis are also found in the region (Aroni et al., 2003). In Peru, the following varieties have been obtained: Yellow Maranganí, Kancolla, Juli White, Cheweca, Witulla, Salcedo-INIA, Iplla-INIA, Quillahuaman-INIA, Camacani I, Camacani II, Huariponcho, Chullpi, Coporaque Red, Ayacuchana-INIA, Huancayo, Hualhuas, Mantaro, Huacataz, Huacariz, Yanamango Pink, Namora, Tahuaco, Yocará, Wilacayuni, Pacus, Junín Pink, Junín White, Acostambo y Ayacuchana White (Mujica et al., 2004; Mujica, 1992). In Ecuador, the following varieties have been obtained: Tunkahuan, Ingapirca, Cochasqui, Imbaya, Chaucha, Tanlahua, Piartal, Porotoc, Chimborazo bitter, Imbabura bitter and Purple (Mujica et al., 2004; Tapia, 1990; Mujica, 1992). According to Peralta (2006) the Tunkahuan variety is effective and is the most planted in the highlands of Ecuador, Peralta also indicates that in 2004 the variety Pata de Venado was released.

CHIA SEEDS

CHEMICAL COMPOSITION

Salvia is a genus of about 900 green shrub-like plants of the Salvia L. family. *Salvia hispanica* L., commonly known as chia, is the representative of the Salvia genus. The chia family is mainly recognized for its high nutritional and therapeutic potential. *S. hispanica* L. is grown in western Mexico to northern Guatemala stretch as an annual plant. It shows optimal development in a warm climate, high rainfall, and temperatures of 15°C–30°C (Coates and Ayerza, 1996; Coates and Ayerza, 1998). The plant attains a maximum height of 1 m. It has opposite leaves, 4–8 cm long and 3–6 cm wide (Nutritional Nutrient Database for Standard Reference, 2011). The chia flowers, purplish-white and sized 3–4 mm, are gathered in whorls on top of shoots. Its fruits (schizocarps) contain numerous oval seeds, which are about 2 mm long. The seeds are mottle-colored with brown, grey, black, and white (Ixtainaa et al., 2008; Ali et al., 2012; Olivos-Lugo et al., 2010). The word 'chia' derives from the Náhuatl word 'Chian', which means 'oily'. Its name was given to the plant by Carl Linnaeus (1707–1778), who discovered the wild-growing plant in the new world and confused it with a native plant from Spain (Edwards, 1819). However, chia comes from Mexico and it was imported to Spain by Hernán Cortés (Ortiz de Montellano, 1978). Chia seed's high nutritional potential is attributed to its seed composition. The seed composition mainly depends on genetic factors and the ecosystems where the plants were grown (Ayerza and Coates, 2011). Chia seeds contain approx. About 16%–26% of protein, 31%–34% of fat, 37%–45% of carbohydrates in total, 23%–35% of total dietary fiber. They are also considered a good source of calcium, phosphorus, potassium, and magnesium. The Vitamins (thiamine, riboflavin, niacin, folic acid, ascorbic acid, and vitamin A) and antioxidant compounds are also very high in chia seeds(Ixtainaa, 2008; Mohd Ali et al., 2012). The energy value of chia seeds is 459–495 kcal/100g (Coates and Ayerza, 1998; Lima et al., 2011). The influence of bioactive compounds in chia seeds is the subject of research conducted in numerous scientific centers. The nutritional properties of chia seeds(high content of polyunsaturated fatty acids, vegetable protein, dietary fiber, vitamins, minerals, and bioactive substances) result in numerous studies on these seeds to prove their therapeutic properties. Antineoplastic, laxative, and analgesic properties are other properties of chia seeds, and they are said to protect the cardiovascular system (Ayerza and Coates, 2005); also, they exhibit anti-inflammatory properties along with controlling lipid metabolism (Brenna et al., 2009; Chicco et al., 2008; Rodea-Gonzáleza et al., 2012), have anti-oxidative properties and increase the performance of athletes (Ulbricht et al., 2009). Anticoagulant and anti-inflammatory effects of chia seeds may help prevent strokes and heart attacks in type-II diabetic patients (Vuksan et al., 2007). An increase of unsaturated fatty acids in plasma blood was also observed in the study of healthy postmenopausal women supplemented with 25 g milled chia seeds per day for seven weeks (Jin et al., 2012). The effect of ingesting chia seeds for a few weeks was examined on many adults. Various studies found no significant reduction in inflammatory markers, body weight, blood pressure, lipid profile, and blood sugar levels. Similar results were obtained in the study conducted with 62 obese women supplemented with 25 g whole or 25 g milled chia seeds (Nieman et al., 2009). However, a reduction in postprandial glycemia in healthy subjects was shown in other studies (Ho et al., 2013; Vuksan et al., 2010; Vuksan et al., 2016). To evaluate the effect of dietary intervention in checking metabolic syndromes, a randomized, double-blind trial was done. This trial conducted on 67 adults found a significant reduction of triacylglycerols, C-reactive protein concentrations, and insulin resistance in a group with a chia-based diet (Guevara-Cruz et al., 2012). It was observed that ingesting 35 g chia flour for 12 weeks decreased total cholesterol level and increased LDL cholesterol (Toscano et al., 2015). Although the presence of many bioactive ingredients in chia seeds contributes to many health benefits, safety, and efficiency of this medicinal food or natural product, they need to be validated by scientific protocols since clinical studies on the safety and efficiency of chia seeds are still limited and those reported have not shown conclusive results (Valdivia-López and Tecante, 2015).

TYPES OF CHIA SEEDS

Chia seeds are grown in a natural environment in both black and white seed forms – the black chia seeds have a veined coloring and are grown in the majority nowadays. White chia seeds are more prominent and are found in much lower percentages.

Farmers separate the white seeds before planting as white seeds result in plants bearing more white seeds to increase the percentage of the harvest of white seeds. Historically farmers were growing white and black chia seeds as different crops. However, over time the white chia production decreased and became mixed with the more commonly produced black chia seeds.

The black chia seeds are a tiny bit higher in antioxidants. Comparatively higher amount of oil (34.66±0.63%) with soya beans 22.43±0.53% is found in black chia seeds. Ash content of black chia seeds was 4.72±0%. As proven by various studies, high concentrations of polyunsaturated fatty acids (α-linoleic acid) and low quantities of primary saturated fatty acids (Taga et al., 1984; Oliveira-Alves et al., 2017; Caruso et al., 2018) are also found in chia seeds. Dietary fiber has become an essential component in the everyday diet because of its various medicinal benefits, such as reducing cholesterolemia, modifying the glycemic and insulinemic responses, changes in intestinal activity (Reyes-Caudillo et al., 2008). As we all know, dietary fiber is a mixture of compounds consisting of cellulose, gums, hemicellulose, and pectic substances that may be associated with lignin. Valdivia-López and Tecante (2015) found that chia seeds had 2.4, 2.5, 8.2, and 9.7 times more fiber per 100 g of the edible portion than wheat, oat, maize, and rice, respectively. It is also found that black chia seeds had a higher content of PDF, ADF., ADL, and hemicellulose (31.18±0.18, 14.83±0.08, 13.19±0.20, 15.94±0.22%, respectively), but a lower content of cellulose (2.87±0.19%). The lignin component supposedly protects unsaturated oils in chia seeds by building a solid and resistant structure and its antioxidants. Due to its bile acids absorbing potential, lignin promotes the hypocholesterolemic effect of fiber intake (Valdivia-López and Tecante, 2015). High neutral detergent fiber (PDF) content (32.18%) indicates the presence of diverse carbohydrates that form the structure of mucilage – a protective layer for the seed embryo that swells in contact with water forming a sticky gelatinous capsule. To attain the desired food product functionality and texture, the utilizable value of mucilage has been growing in recent years. The mucilage can be used as a fat substitute in many food products such as in cakes, ice creams as an emulsifier and stabilizer, in bread as a fat replacer (Punia and Dhull, 2019). The high fiber content determined in black chia seed samples indicates that the consumption of these seeds as a food component could provide both nutritional and health-promoting standpoints. The total protein content determined in black chia seeds (25.04±0.20%) is following the results of a study conducted by Žilić (2011) and Valdivia-López and Tecante (2015). Water-soluble albumins had the highest content of all soluble proteins in black chia seeds, and they also had the highest content of globulins 14.64±0.07% d.m. and NSI 58.48±0.27% of total protein. Gliadins soluble in ethanol had the lowest content of all soluble proteins in both investigated species (0.94±0% in chia). The content of glutenins soluble in borate buffer was slightly higher (2.72±0% in chia). Chia seeds contain essential amino acids, unlike most vegetable protein sources that lack two or more amino acids, so they have a better protein quality than cereals and the other seeds (Nitrayova et al., 2014; Valdivia-López and Tecante, 2015). The total phenolic compounds value in black chia seed extracts amounted to 1201.94±16.29 mg GAE/kg; that is, the content was slightly higher than the one reported by Reyes-Caudillo et al. (2008), who found that the total content of phenolics of chia seeds in crude extracts was 0.9211±0.040 mg GAE/g for Jalisco and 0.8800±0.008 mg GAE/g for Sinaloa variety of chia (i.e., 921.1 and 880.0 mg GAE/kg). The total flavonoids content was detected in black chia seeds (233.98±8.42 mg CE/kg).

Nutritional values are similar in black and white chia seeds; some constituents like protein content. Scientists found that protein content in black chia seeds is 16.9% and fiber content is 32.6%, and in white chia seeds, the protein content is reported to be 16.5% and the fiber content 32.4%. The difference is seen in morphological features such as – white seeds are comparatively larger, thicker, and broader. Interestingly, when black chia seeds are cultivated, around 5% to 8% of white chia seeds are grown simultaneously. Cultivating only white chia seeds gives white chia seeds only.

The plant produces black and white seeds. Chia seeds are generally tiny, approximately 2 mm long, 1–1.5 mm wide, and thicker than 1.0 mm, flat and oval-shaped. Black-colored chia seeds, which are more common, only slightly differ from the white seeds by their morphology; white seeds are more prominent, thicker, and broader than the black seeds. Their composition is similar; it is reported that the average moisture content of black and white seeds is around 6%, one-third of the material in the oil; however, some authors report deviations in protein and fatty acid composition of both seed varieties (Ixtaina et al., 2008; Capitani et al., 2012). In human nutrition, chia seeds can be used as whole, milled, or ground. Oil extracted from chia seeds can also be used in food (Capitani et al., 2012; Reyes-Caudillo et al., 2008). Recently, several evaluations of chia's properties and possible uses have been performed. The high content of oil, from 30 to more than 40%, of which 60% represents (omega) ω-3 alpha-linolenic acid and 20% (omega) ω-6 linoleic acid (Ali et al., 2012). Both essential fatty acids are associated with various benefits to consumer health, including preventing cardiovascular diseases and various diseases such as type 2 diabetes and cancer and protecting against Alzheimer's (Alfredo et al., 2009). Chia crop has undoubtedly a high potential to become a part of a modern balanced diet, not only because of its oil quality but also due to the presence of natural antioxidants, protein (15%–20%), carbohydrates (26%–41%), high dietary fiber (18%–30%), ash (4%–5%), minerals, vitamins, and dry matter (90%–93%). Since chia is identified as a species with oil production potential, many oil extraction methods had been utilized. Variations in the extraction conditions, method, and solvent choice resulted in differences in the oil yield, quality of fatty acids, fatty acid contents, total dietary fibers, and antioxidant content. However, oil extraction of chia produces a subfraction with relatively high dietary fiber content rich in polyphenols, possibly involved in high antioxidant activity, and compounds conferring functional characteristics with food system applications (Fernandes and de las Mercedes Salas-Mellado, 2017). Extraction of oil from chia seeds has been traditionally performed by cold pressing technique. This method is undoubtedly featured by better preserving antioxidant contents such as quercetin and myricetin than solvent extraction (Capitani et al., 2012). However, the recovery of oil yield is relatively low (Ixtaina et al., 2008). The Soxhlet method using n-hexane has been most widely applied among solvent extraction techniques even though it is not preferable to other methods, which do not involve aggressive organic solvents (Azmir et al., 2014).

THE THERAPEUTIC VALUE OF CHIA AND QUINOA SEEDS

Chia seeds possess various therapeutic values as well. Such as cardio-protective effects were analyzed by Munoz et al. (2012). The constituent found in chia seeds, α-linolenic acid, plays a significant role in forming some vital biochemical components such as leukotrienes and thromboxanes, which are supposed to be connected to numerous physiological functions in the human body (Ullah et al., 2016). Moreover, the ω-3 fatty acid compound has the capability of blocking calcium and sodium channels dysfunctions (which can cause hypertension), improve the parasympathetic tone, and protect ventricular arrhythmia (Ullah et al., 2016). Furthermore, eating chia seeds in the pregnancy helps in developing the retina and brain of the fetus (Table 6.1).

Adding to it, incorporating dietary fiber and a-linolenic fatty acids into the diet makes chia a prime contender in regulating diabetes. A study conducted by Vuksan and co-workers demonstrated that supplementing 37 g/day of Salba chia to a diet improves significant risk factors in type 2 diabetes and suggests its cardioprotective potential while maintaining a healthy weight. A subsequent follow-up study done by the same group of researchers demonstrated that if Salba-chia is added to a meal, it acutely reduces postprandial glycemia and prolongs satiety. Further investigations demonstrated that if Salba-chia is added to the diet for six months and a calorie-restricted diet is maintained(in addition to standard medical care), significant but small weight loss obese participants with type 2 diabetes is observed (Vuksan et al., 2017). Salba-chia appears to potentially convert glucose into a slow-release carbohydrate and affect satiety value to a much greater extent than flaxseeds, possibly due to the higher fiber viscosity. This fact was supported by a study conducted on 15 healthy participants (M/F: 5/10; age: 23.9 ± three years; BMI: 22.2 ± 0.8 kg/m^2) to whom 50 g glucose challenge was given randomly, alone, or supplemented with either 25 g ground Salba-chia or 31.5 g flax, on three separate occasions. Then their blood samples were taken for analyzing glucose content, and after fasting, satiety ratings were collected over 2 hours postprandially. Also, rheological methods were used for assessing *in vitro* viscosity of the beverages.

Salba chia appeared to differentially alter carbohydrate metabolism and satiety and have a more substantial effect than flaxseeds. The blood glucose iAUC (Incremental Area Under the Curve) observed a 39% reduction for ground Salba-chia which is in line with the reductions from previous studies of 35% and 42% vs. control at a comparable dose of 24 g. Interestingly, ground flax shows contrasting results in affecting postprandial glycemia. The findings of various researchers suggest that the criteria for the selection of seeds must also include their rheological properties rather than their absolute fiber content. Namely, viscosity is considered a measure of the fiber's contribution to viscosity development, independent of fiber concentration (Vuksan et al., 2017). The consumption of chia flour consistently may be proven to decrease the blood pressure in hypertensive individuals, even in patients who were on medications previously, like the patients not using medications. Despite the reduction in lipid peroxidation as the effect of chia, there was no verification of the fact that it is because of the antioxidant content present in seeds. The effectiveness of milled and whole chia seeds in altering disease risk factors in overweight,

TABLE 6.1
The Therapeutic Properties of Chia Seeds

Decreased body weight in the group consuming chia flour, a more significant decrease in obese people, no different from the placebo group. Reduced total cholesterol and increased LDL cholesterol in the supplemented group.	Tavares Toscano L., Leite Tavares R., Oliveira Silva C.S., Silva A.S.: Chia induces clinically discrete weight loss and improves lipid profile only in altered previous values. *Nutr Hosp* 2015; 31(3):1176-1182.
Chia seeds and oil reduced oxidative stress *in vivo* by improving the antioxidant status and lipid peroxidation in diet-induced obese rats.	Marineli R.S., Lenquiste S.A., Moraes E.A., Maróstica M.R.: Antioxidant potential of dietary chia seed and oil (*Salvia hispanica* L.) in diet-induced obese rats. *Food Res Int* 2015;76(3):666-674.
Reduced concentration of triacylglycerols and increased content of α-linolenic acid in the serum in HD-cd group. Chia seed oil may have a protective effect on blood vessels.	Sierra L., Roco J., Alarcon G., Medina M., Nieuwenhove C.V., Peral de Bruno M., Jerez S.: Dietary intervention with *Salvia hispanica* (Chia) oil improves vascular function in rabbits under hypercholesterolaemic conditions. *J Functional Foods* 2015; 14:641-649.
The blood test showed reduced postprandial glycemia.	Ho H., Lee A.S., Jovanovski E., Jenkins A.L., Desouza R., Vuksan V.: Effect of whole and ground Salba seeds (*Salvia Hispanica* L.) on postprandial glycemia healthy volunteers: a randomized controlled, dose-response trial. *Eur J Clin Nutr* 2013;67(2):105-110.
No influence of [whole/ground] seeds on inflammatory markers, blood pressure, body composition. Increased concentration of α-linolenic and eicosapentaenoic acids in the blood serum of obese women consuming ground seeds vs. the control group and the group consuming whole chia seeds.	. Nieman D.C., Gillitt N., Jin F., Henson D.A., Kennerly K., Shanely R.A., Ore B., Su M., Schwartz S.: Chia seed supplementation and disease risk factors in overweight women: a metabolomics investigation. *J Altern Complement Med* 2012;18(7):700-708.
Reduced concentration of triacylglycerols, CRP and insulin resistance in the supplemented group.	Guevara-Cruz M., Tovar A.R., Aguilar-Salinas C.A., Medina-Vera I., Gil-Zenteno L., Hernández-Viveros I., López-Romero P., Ordaz-Nava G., Canizales-Quinteros S., Guillen Pineda L.E., Torres N.: A dietary pattern including nopal, chia seed, soy protein, and oat reduces serum triglycerides and glucose intolerance in patients with metabolic syndrome. *J Nutr* 2012; 142(1):64-69.
Increased concentration of α-linolenic and eicosapentaenoic acids in the serum of women supplemented with ground chia seeds.	Jin F., Nieman D.C., Sha W., Xie G., Qiu Y., Jia W.: Supplementation of milled chia seeds increases plasma ALA and EPA in postmenopausal women. *Plant Foods Hum Nutr* 2012; 67:105-110.
Postprandial glycemia was significantly reduced in comparison with the control group.	Vuksan V., Jenkins A.L., Dias A.G., Lee A.S., Jovanovski E., Rogovik A.L., Hanna A.: Reduction in postprandial glucose excursion and prolongation of satiety: possible explanation of the long-term effects of whole grain Salba (*Salvia Hispanica* L.). *Eur J Clin Nutr* 2010; 64(4):436-438.

(Continued)

TABLE 6.1 (*Continued*)
The Therapeutic Properties of Chia Seeds

Increased concentration of α-linolenic acid in the serum of the group under study vs. placebo. No influence of seeds on inflammatory markers, blood pressure, body composition.	Nieman D.C., Cayea E.J., Austin M.D., Henson D.A., McAnulty S.R., Jin F.: Chia seed does not promote weight loss or alter disease risk factors in overweight adults. *Nutr Res* 2009;29(6):414-418.
No influence on IgE concentration in the serum, body weight, and thymus weight.	Fernandez I., Vidueiros S.M., Ayerza R., Coates W., Pallaro A.: Impact of chia (*Salvia hispanica* L.) on the immune system: a preliminary study. *Proc Nutr Soc* 2008;67(OCE):12.
Reduced triglyceride concentration in the serum of T2 rats and increased HDL content in the serum of T3 rats compared to the control group. Increased concentration of fatty acids 18: 3n–3, 20: 5n–3, and 22: 6n–3 in the serum of T2-T3 rats compared to the control group.	Ayerza R. & Coates W.: Effect of dietary alpha-linolenic fatty acid derived from chia when fed as ground seed, whole seed, and oil on rat plasma lipid content and fatty acid composition. *Ann Nutr Metab* 2007; 51(1):27-34.
Reduced systolic blood pressure and CRP concentration, a double increase in the concentration of α-linolenic and eicosapentaenoic acids in the serum of *Salvia hispanica* patients supplemented with ground chia seeds compared to the control group.	Vuksan V., Whitham D., Sievenpiper J.L., Jenkins A.L., Rogovik A.L., Bazinet R.P., Vidgen E., Hanna A.: Supplementation of conventional therapy with the novel grain Salba (L.) improves major and emerging cardiovascular risk factors in type 2 diabetes: Results of a randomized controlled trial. *Diabetes Care* 2007; 30(11):2804-2810.

postmenopausal women was studied using a metabolomics approach. In total, 62 overweight (body–mass index 25 kg/m^2 and higher), nondiseased, nonsmoking, postmenopausal women, ages 49–75 years have been included. The study was performed employing analysis based on the 56 subjects who completed all phases of the study – diet records and questionnaire responses to assess potential adverse effects and adherence to the supplementation regimen were administered as a prestudy, and after 5- and 10-week supplementation.

Quinoa's properties, such as its high nutritional value, therapeutic properties, and being gluten-free, benefit several lactose intolerant consumers, including children, the elderly, high-performance athletes, osteoporosis-prone women, anemia, patients with diabetes, obesity, or celiac disease (Bhargava and others, 2006; Vega-Gálvez and others, 2010). Although there are not many reports available on clinical trials animal and human beings on the therapeutic potential of quinoa, many studies are indicating various health benefits associated with quinoa consumption. In a nutrition study conducted on children, mainly boys aged 4–5 years coming from low-income families living in Ecuador, it was found that the formulation of infant food with quinoa (approx.100 g twice per day for 15 days) significantly brought an increase in plasma IGF-1 levels, when IGF-1 levels were unaffected in the control group. IGF-1 is a hepatic peptide that promotes growth with an increase in body weight and bone length. IGF-1 has been observed as a marker of malnutrition. The high digestibility

(95.3%) of quinoa was attributed to its complete amino acid profile, which was higher than that of 5 commercially available infant foods derived from milk and soy. Quinoa formulated Infant food provides sufficient protein and other essential nutrients crucial for reducing child malnutrition (Ruales and others, 2002).

Clinical Human trials evaluated the use of quinoa seeds as a gluten-free alternative to cereal grains among celiac patients. Selected 19 celiac patients consumed 50 g quinoa daily for 42 days. Various gastrointestinal parameters (villus height: crypt depth, surface-enterocyte cell height, and the number of intraepithelial lymphocytes and lipid levels(serum) were evaluated before and after the intervention. The gastrointestinal parameters improved following the quinoa diet. At the same time, serum lipid levels remained within a normal range, with a slight reduction in lipid profile values (LDL, HDL, and total triglycerides) (Zevallos and others, 2014). This study was also endorsed by human trials done by Farinazzi-Machado et al. in 2012. They confirmed that daily consumption of quinoa cereal bars for 30 days resulted in low values for lipid profile. Also, body weight, blood glucose, and blood pressure levels were decreased in 18–45 years.

In a double-blinded human clinical trial among postmenopausal women with excess weight, quinoa flake consumption (25 g/d for four weeks) also modulated metabolic parameters posttreatment compared to baseline and serum triglycerides (111.3 ± 36 to 106.8 ± 3.5 mg/dL) and TBAR values (3.07 ± 0.5 to 2.99 ± 0.6 μmol/L (TBARs are substances produced in response to lipid peroxidation-induced oxidative stress) were both significantly reduced. Furthermore, quinoa intervention nonsignificantly reduced total cholesterol (192 ± 34 to 182 ± 18 mg/dL) and LDL-cholesterol (130 ± 35 to 120 ± 25 mg/dL), while glutathione (GSH, a marker of antioxidant defense) was increased (1.79 ± 0.3 to 1.92 ± 0.3 mmol/L). Similar decreases in lipid profile and TBAR values were observed in a parallel intervention group given corn flakes instead of quinoa (De Carvalho and others, 2014).

Although the antidiabetic effects of quinoa have not been studied in humans, co-administration of quinoa seeds (310 g/kg feed for 150 days) resulted in reduced glucose levels in plasma and oxidative stress in rats fed on 31% fructose diet compared to the control group (Pasko and others,_2010a,b). Also, it was observed that phytochemically enriched products derived from quinoa seeds (described in detail below) significantly lowered fasting blood glucose, adiposity, and cholesterol *levels in vivo* (Foucault and others, 2011, 2014; Graf and others, 2014).

The evidence from the studies available for quinoa's health benefits warrants future studies on this crop's role in treating and preventing human disorders/diseases. Controlled and Randomized trials are the gold standard for determining the effect of diet on health outcomes. However, certain factors are considered crucial for determining trial outcomes, such as optimal study design and length of the study.

It is essential to utilize quinoa products with well-characterized and standardized phytochemical contents within clinical intervention studies to link observed effects to specific constituents. Previous clinical studies collectively suggest that the significant cholesterol-lowering and antioxidant properties of quinoa were due to its proteins, fiber, vitamins (tocopherols and carotenoids), minerals (iron, zinc, magnesium), saponins, phytosterols, phytoecdysteroids, and phenolics content (Rules and others, 2002; Farinazzi-Machado and others, 2012; De Carvalho and others, 2014; Zevallos and others, 2014). Not to mention, other constituents like phytochemicals naming polyunsaturated fatty acids and betalains also have a significant role. Individual quinoa constituents also positively interact with each other, which leads to enhanced bioactivity through a phenomenon called synergistic or potentiation effect (Schmidt and others, 2008). Some scientists claim that whole grains have shown that their health benefits are likely due to the 'whole-grain package' effect rather than every single constituent of the grain (McKeown and others, 2013). A single serving of 40 g quinoa will deliver a large portion of the Recommended Daily Allowance (RDA) of essential nutrients and health-beneficial compounds to the consumer Keeping into view the complex nature of quinoa's phytochemical profile; it is essential to take a note of the 'whole-grain package' hypothesis before designing or analyzing the results of future clinical trials/studies.

Patient perspective/compliance is yet another factor to consider when conducting human trials. Quinoa products used in human studies should appeal to consumers, like packaged snacks and energy bars. Plant lignins result in compounds like enterodiol and enterolactone from the metabolism by gut microbiota. Several variables affect the efficiency of gut microbiota conversion of lignans to enterolignans (intestinal integrity, stress, genetics, antibiotic intake) (van Dam and Hu, 2008; De Carvalho and others, 2014).

BIBLIOGRAPHY

Abugoch James, L. E. (2009). Chapter 1 Quinoa (*Chenopodium quinoa Willd.*). *Adv Food Nutr Res* 1:1–31.

Alfredo, V. O., Gabriel, R. R., Luis, C. G., and David, B. A. (2009). Physicochemical properties of a fibrous fraction from chia (*Salvia hispanica L.*). *LWT-Food Sci Technol* 42:168–173.

Ali, N. M., Yeap, S. K., Ho, W. Y., Beh, B. K., Tan, S. W., and Tan, S. G. (2012). The promising future of chia, *Salvia hispanica* L. *J Biomed Biotechnol* 2012:1–9. Article ID 171956. https://doi.org/10.1155/2012/171956.

Aroni, J. C., Aroni, G., Quispe, R., and Bonifacio, A. (2003). *Catálogo de Quinua Real. Fundación PROINPA. SIBTA – SINARGEAA. Fundación Altiplano. Fundación Mcknight.* COSUDE, La Paz, 51.

Ayerza R. and Coates W. (2005). *Chia: Rediscovering an Ancient Crop of the Aztecs.* University of Arizona Press, Tuscon.

Ayerza R. and Coates W. (2011). Protein content, oil content and fatty acid profiles as potential criteria to determine the origin of commercially grown chia (*Salvia hispanica* L.). *Ind Crop Prod* 34:1366–1371.

Azmir, J., Zaidul, I. S. M., Rahman, M. M., Sharif, K. M., Sahena, F., Jahurul, M. H. A., and Mohamed, A. (2014). Optimization of oil yield of *Phaleria macrocarpa* seed using response surface methodology and its fatty acids constituents. *Ind Crops Prod* 52:405–412.

Bazile, D., Jacobsen, S. E., and Verniau, A. (2016). The global expansion of quinoa: Trends and limits. *Front Plant Sci* 7:622.

Bertero, H. D., De la Vega, A. J., Correa, G., Jacobsen, S. E., and Mujica, A. (2004). Genotype and genotype-by-environment interaction effects for grain yield and grain size of quinoa (Chenopodium quinoa Willd.) as revealed by pattern analysis of international multi-environment trials. *Field Crops Res* 89:299–318.

Bhargava, A., Shukla, S., and Ohri, D. (2006). *Chenopodium quinoa* – an Indian perspective. *Industrial Crops and Products* 23:73–87.

Biodiversity International. (2007). Quinoa: A delicate balancing act. Biodiversity International Annual Report 2006, pp. 17–19.

Boesewinkel, F. D. and Bouman, F. (1984). The seed: Structure. *Embryology Angiosperms* 1:567–610.

Bouman, F. (1984). The ovule. *Embryology Angiosperms* 1:123–157.

Brenna, J. T., Salem Jr, N., Sinclair, A. J., and Cunnane, S. C. (2009). α-Linolenic acid supplementation and conversion to n-3 long-chain polyunsaturated fatty acids in humans. *Prostaglandins Leukot Essent Fatty Acids* 80:85–91.

Caruso, M. C., Favati, F., Di Cairano, M., Galgano, F., Labella, R., Scarpa, T., and Condelli, N. (2018). Shelf-life evaluation and nutraceutical properties of chia seeds from a recent long-day flowering genotype cultivated in Mediterranean area. *LWT* 87:400–405.

Chicco, A. G., D'Alessandro, M. E., Hein, G. J., Oliva, M. E., and Lombardo, Y. B. (2008). Dietary chia seed (*Salvia hispanica* L.) rich in α-linolenic acid improves adiposity and normalises hypertriacylglycerolaemia and insulin resistance in dyslipaemic rats. *Br J Nutr* 101:41–50.

Coates, W. (1996). Production potential of chia in northwestern Argentina. *Ind Crops Prod* 5:229–233.

Coates, W. and Ayerza, R. (1998). Commercial production of chia in Northwestern Argentina. *J Am Oil Chemists' Soc* 75:1417–1420.

Cusack, D. F. (1984). Quinua-grain of the Incas. *Ecologist* 14:21–31.

De Carvalho, F. G., Ovidio, P. P., Padovan, G. J., Jordao Junior, A. A., Marchini, J. S., Navarro, A. M. (2014). Metabolic parameters of postmenopausal women after quinoa or corn flakes intake – a prospective and double-blind study. *Int J Food Sci Nutr* 65(3):380–385.

Edwards S. S. (1819). Salvia hispanica, Spanish Sage. *Botanical Register* 5:359.

Farinazzi-Machado, F. M. V., Barbalho, S. M., Oshiiwa, M., Goulart, R., and Pessan Junior, O. (2012). Use of cereal bars with quinoa (Chenopodium quinoa W.) to reduce risk factors related to cardiovascular diseases. *Cienc Technol Aliment Campinas* 32(3):239–244.

Fernandes, S. S., and de las Mercedes Salas-Mellado, M. (2017). Addition of chia seed mucilage for reduction of fat content in bread and cakes. *Food Chem* 227:237–244.

Foucault, A.-S., Even, P., Lafont, R., Dioh, W., Veillet, S., Tomé, D., Huneau, J.-F., Hermier, D., and Quignard-Boulangé, A. (2014). Quinoa extract enriched in 20-hydroxyecdysone affects energy homeostasis and intestinal fat absorption in mice fed a high-fat diet. *Physiology & Behavior* 128:226–231. doi:10.1016/j.physbeh.2014.02.002

Fuentes, F. F., Bazile, D., Bhargava, A., and Martinez, E. A. (2012). Implications of farmers' seed exchanges for on-farm conservation of quinoa, as revealed by its genetic diversity in Chile. *J Agri Sci* 150:702–716.

Galwey, N. W., Leakey, C. L. A., Price, K. R., and Fenwick, G. R. (1989). Chemical composition and nutritional characteristics of quinoa (Chenopodium quinoa Willd.). *Food Sci Nutr* 42:245–261.

Graf, B. L., Poulev, A., Kuhn, P., Grace, M. H., Lila, M. A., and Raskin, I. (2014). Quinoa seeds leach phytoecdysteroids and other compounds with anti-diabetic properties. Food Chem 163:178–185. doi:10.1016/j.foodchem.2014.04.088

Guevara-Cruz, M., Tovar, A. R., Aguilar-Salinas, C. A., Medina-Vera, I., Gil-Zenteno, L., Hernández-Viveros, I., and Torres, N. (2012). A dietary pattern including nopal, chia seed, soy protein, and oat reduces serum triglycerides and glucose intolerance in patients with metabolic syndrome. *J Nutr* 142:64–69.

Herencia, L. I., Al!ıa, M., Gonzalez, J. A., and Urbano, P. (1999). Cultivo de la quinoa (Chenopodium Quinoa Willd.) en la region! Centro. (The culture of quinoa in the central region). *Vida Rural*, Ano VI(87):28–33.

Ho, H., Lee, A. S., Jovanovski, E., Jenkins, A. L., Desouza, R., and Vuksan, V. (2013). Effect of whole and ground Salba seeds (*Salvia hispanica* L.) on postprandial glycemia in healthy volunteers: A randomized controlled, dose-response trial. *Eur J Clin Nutr* 67:786–788.

Ixtaina, V. Y., Nolascoa, S. M., and Tomas, M. C. (2008). Physical properties of chia (*Salvia hispanica* L.) seeds. *Ind Crops Prod* 28:286–293.

Jacobsen, S. E. (2011). The situation for quinoa and its production in southern Bolivia: From economic success to environmental disaster. *J Agron Crop Sci* 197(5):390–399.

Jin, F., Nieman, D. C., Sha, W., Xie, G., Qiu, Y., and Jia, W. (2012). Supplementation of milled chia seeds increases plasma ALA and EPA in postmenopausal women. *Plant Foods Human Nutr* 67:105–110.

Kozioł, M. J. (1992). Chemical composition and nutritional evaluation of quinoa (Chenopodium quinoa Willd.). *J Food Compos Anal* 5:35–68.

Lescano, J. L. (1989). Recursos fitogenéticos altoandinos y bancos de germoplas. In: *Curso: "Cultivos altoandinos"*. Potosí, Bolivia, 1–18.

Lima, D. M., Padovani, R. M., Rodriguez-Amaya, D. B., Farfán, J. A., Nonato, C. T., and De Lima, M. T. (2011). Table Brazilian food composition. NEPA/UNICAMP, 4th ed. NEPA – UNICAMP, Campinas, 161.

McElhinny, E., Peralta, E., Mazon, N., Danial, D. L., Thiele, G., and Lindhout, P. (2007). Aspects of participatory plant breeding for quinoa in marginal areas of Ecuador. *Euphytica* 153:373–384.

McKeown, N. M., Jacques, P. F., Seal, C. J., de Vries, J., Jonnalagadda, S. S., Clemens, R., Webb, D., Murphy, L. A., van Klinken, J. W., Topping, D., Murray, R., Degeneffe, D., and Marquart, L. F. (2013). Whole grains and health: from theory to practice – highlights of the Grains for Health Foundation's Whole Grains Summit 2012. J Nutr 143(5): 744S–758S.

Mohd Ali, N., Yeap, S. K., Ho, W. Y., Beh, B. K., Tan, S. W., and Tan, S. G. (2012). The promising future of chia, *Salvia hispanica* L. *J Biomed Biotechnol* 2012.

Mujica, A. (1992). Andean grains and legumes. In: *Crops Marginalized: Another Perspective of 1492*. J. Hernandez, J. Bermejo, and J. Leon (Eds.). Organization of United Nations Food and Agriculture FAO, Rome, 129–146.

Mujica, A. (1994). Andean grains and legumes. J. E. H. Bermujo and J. Leon (Eds.). *Neglected Crops* 1492:131–148.

Mujica, A., Cahahua, A., and Saravia, R. (2004). Agronomía de la quinua. In: *Quinua: Ancestral cultivo andino, alimento del presente y futuro*. A. Mujica, S. Jacobsen, J. Izquierdo, and J. P. Marathee (Eds.). FAO, UNA, CIP, Santiago, Chile, 26–59.

Muñoz, L. A., Cobos, A., Diaz, O., and Aguilera, J. M. (2012). Chia seeds: Microstructure, mucilage extraction and hydration. *J Food Eng* 108:216–224.

Nieman, D. C., Cayea, E. J., Austin, M. D., Henson, D. A., McAnulty, S. R., and Jin, F. (2009). Chia seed does not promote weight loss or alter disease risk factors in overweight adults. *Nutrition Res* 29:414–418.

Nikolić, V., Žilić, S., Simić, M., and Perić, V. (2020). Black soya bean and black chia seeds as a source of nutrients and bioactive compounds with health benefits. *Food and Feed Res* 47:2.

Nitrayova, S., Brestenský, M., Heger, J., Patras, P., Rafay, J., and Sirotkin, A. (2014). Amino acids and fatty acids profile of chia (Salvia hispanica L.) and flax (Linum usitatissimum L.) seed. *Potravinarstvo*, 8(1):72–76. https://doi.org/10.5219/332

Oliveira-Alves, S. C., Vendramini-Costa, D. B., Cazarin, C. B. B., Júnior, M. R. M., Ferreira, J. P. B., Silva, A. B., and Bronze, M. R. (2017). Characterization of phenolic compounds in chia (*Salvia hispanica* L.) seeds, fiber flour and oil. *Food Chem* 232:295–305.

Olivos-Lugo, B. L., Valdivia-López, M. Á., and Tecante, A. (2010). Thermal and physicochemical properties and nutritional value of the protein fraction of Mexican chia seed (*Salvia hispanica* L.). *Food Sci Technol Int* 16:89–96.

Ormachea, E. and Quispe, D. (1993). Evaluation of parasitoids of the "quinoa moth" Eurysacca melanocampta, in Cusco. XXXV National Convention of Entomology.

Ortiz de Montellano, B. R. (1978). Aztec cannibalism: An ecological necessity? *Science* 200:611–617.

Oshodi, H. N., Ogungbenle, M. O., and Oladimeji, A. A. (1999). Chemical composition, nutritionally valuable minerals and functional properties of benniseed (Sesamum radiatum), pearl millet (Pennisetum typhoides) and quinoa (Chenopodium quinoa) flours. *Int J Food Sci Nutr* 50:325–331.

Paśko, P., Bartoń, H., Zagrodzki, P., Gorinstein, S., Fołta, M., and Zachwieja, Z. (2009). Anthocyanins, total polyphenols and antioxidant activity in amaranth and quinoa seeds and sprouts during their growth. *Food Chem* 115:994–998.

Pasko, P., Zagrodzki, P., Barton, H., Chlopicka, J., and Gorinstein, S. (2010a). Effect of quinoa seeds (Chenopodiumquinoa) in diet on some biochemical parameters and essential elements in blood of high fructose-fed rats. *Plant Foods Hum Nutr* 65:333-338.

Pasko, P., Barton, H., Zagrodzki, P., Izewska, A., Krosniak, M., et al. (2010b). Effect of diet supplemented with quinoa seeds on oxidative status in plasma and selected tissues of high fructose-fed rats. *Plant Foods Hum Nutr* 65:146-151.

Peñas, E., Uberti, F., di Lorenzo, C., Ballabio, C., Brandolini, A., and Restani, P. (2014). Biochemical and immunochemical evidences supporting the inclusion of quinoa (Chenopodium quinoa Willd.) as a gluten-free ingredient. *Plant Foods Human Nutr* 69:297–303.

Peralta, E. (2006). Los cultivos Andinos en el Ecuador. Bancos de germoplasma, Fitomejoramiento y Usos: pasado, presente y futuro. In: *Resúmenes XII Congreso Internacional de Cultivos Andinos.* A. Estrella, M. Batallas, E. Peralta and N. Mazón (Eds). Quito, Ecuador.

Perreault, T. (2013). Dispossession by accumulation? Mining, water and the nature of enclosure on the Bolivian altiplano. *Antipode* 45:1050–1069.

Punia, S. and Dhull, S. B. (2019). Chia seed (*Salvia hispanica* L.) mucilage (a heteropolysaccharide): Functional, thermal, rheological behaviour and its utilization. *Int J Biol Macromol* 140:1084–1090.

Repo-Carrasco, R., Espinoza, C., and Jacobsen, S. E. (2003). Nutritional value and use of the Andean crops quinoa (Chenopodium quinoa) and kañiwa (Chenopodium pallidicaule). *Food Rev Int* 19:179–189.

Reyes-Caudillo, E., Tecante, A., and Valdivia-López, M. A. (2008). Dietary fibre content and antioxidant activity of phenolic compounds present in Mexican chia (*Salvia hispanica* L.) seeds. *Food Chem* 107:656–663.

Robards, A. W. and Humpherson, P. G. (1967). Phytoferritin in plastids of the cambial zone of willow. *Planta* 76:169–178.

Rodea-González, D. A., Cruz-Olivares, J., Román-Guerrero, A., Rodríguez-Huezo, M. E., Vernon-Carter, E. J., and Pérez-Alonso, C. (2012). Spray-dried encapsulation of chia essential oil (*Salvia hispanica* L.) in whey protein concentrate-polysaccharide matrices. *J Food Eng* 111:102–109.

Ruales, J. and Nair, B. M. (1993). Content of fat, vitamins and minerals in quinoa (Chenopodium quinoa, Willd) seeds. *Food Chem* 48:131–136.

Ruales, J., De Grijalva, Y., Lopez-Jaramillo, P., and Nair, B. M. (2002). The nutritional quality of infant food from quinoa and its effect on the plasma level of insulin-like growth factor-1 (IGF-1) in undernourished children. Int *J Food Sci Nutr* 53:143–154.

Ruiz, K. B., Biondi, S., Oses, R., Acuña-Rodríguez, I. S., Antognoni, F., Martinez-Mosqueira, E. A., and Molina-Montenegro, M. A. (2014). Quinoa biodiversity and sustainability for food security under climate change. A review. *Agron Sust Dev* 34:349–359.

Schmidt, B., Ribnicky, D., Poulev, A., Logendra, S., Cefalu, W. T., and Raskin, I. (2008). A natural history of botanical therapeutics. *Metabolism* 57:S3–S9.

Taga, M. S., Miller, E. E., and Pratt, D. E. (1984). Chia seeds as a source of natural lipid antioxidants. *J Am Oil Chem Soc* 61:928–931.

Tapia, M. (1990). *Cultivos Andinos Subexplotados.* FAO, Roma, 204 pp.

Tapia, M. (1997). *Under- exploited Andean Crops and their Contribution to Food.* FAO Regional Office for Latin America and the Caribbean, Santiago.

Toscano, L. T., Toscano, L. T., Tavares, R. L., da Silva, C. S. O., and Silva, A. S. (2015). Chia induces clinically discrete weight loss and improves lipid profile only in altered previous values. *Hosp Nutr* 31:1176–1182.

Ulbricht, C., Chao, W., Nummy, K., Rusie, E., Tanguay-Colucci, S., Iannuzzi, C. M., and Weissner, W. (2009). Chia (*Salvia hispanica*): A systematic review by the natural standard research collaboration. *Rev Recent Clin Trials* 4:168–174.

Ullah, R., Nadeem, M., Khalique, A., Imran, M., Mehmood, S., Javid, A., and Hussain, J. (2016). Nutritional and therapeutic perspectives of chia (*Salvia hispanica* L.): A review. *J Food Sci Technol* 53:1750–1758.

Valdivia-López, M. Á. and Tecante, A. (2015). Chia (*Salvia hispanica*): A review of native Mexican seed and its nutritional and functional properties. *Adv Food Nutr Res* 75:53–75.

Valencia-Chamorro, S. A., ed. (2003). Quinoa. In *Encyclopedia of Food Science and Nutrition*. 2nd edition. Academic Press.

van Dam R. M., Hu, F. B. (2008). Are alkylresorcinols accurate biomarkers for whole grain intake? *Am J Clin Nutr* 87:797–798.

Vega-Gálvez, A., Miranda, M., Vergara, J., Uribe, E., Puente, L., and Martínez, E. A. (2010). Nutrition facts and functional potential of quinoa (Chenopodium quinoa willd.), an ancient Andean grain: A review. *J Sci Food Agri* 90:2541–2547.

Vuksan, V., Choleva, L., Jovanovski, E., Jenkins, A. L., Au-Yeung, F., Dias, A. G., and Duvnjak, L. (2017). Comparison of flax (*Linum usitatissimum*) and Salba-chia (*Salvia hispanica* L.) seeds on postprandial glycemia and satiety in healthy individuals: A randomized, controlled, crossover study. *Eur J Clin Nutr* 71:234–238.

Vuksan, V., Jenkins, A. L., Dias, A. G., Lee, A. S., Jovanovski, E., Rogovik, A. L., and Hanna, A. (2010). Reduction in postprandial glucose excursion and prolongation of satiety: Possible explanation of the long-term effects of whole grain Salba (*Salvia hispanica* L.). *Eur J Clin Nutr* 64:436–438.

Vuksan, V., Whitham, D., Sievenpiper, J. L., Jenkins, A. L., Rogovik, A. L., Bazinet, R. P., and Hanna, A. (2007). Supplementation of conventional therapy with the Novel Grain Salba (*Salvia hispanica* L.) improves major and emerging cardiovascular risk factors in Type 2 diabetes: Results of a randomized controlled trial. *Diabetes Care* 30:2804–2810.

Zevallos, V. F., Herencia, L. I., Chang, F., Donnelly, S., Ellis, H. J., and Ciclitira, P. J. (2014). Gastrointestinal effects of eating quinoa (Chenopodium quinoa Willd.) in celiac patients. *Am J Gastroenterol* 109:270–278.

Žilić, S. (2011). Wheat gluten: Composition and health effects. In: *Gluten: Sources, composition and health effects*. Dane B. Walter (Ed). Nova Science Publisher, Inc., Hauppauge, NY, 71–86.

7 Effect of Processing on Nutritional Properties of Chia and Quinoa Seeds

Chia is an annual herbaceous plant with curative properties of the well-known culinary and medicinal herb *Salvia officinalis* (Dweck, 2005). Nowadays, some species are still used worldwide for their nutritional properties and beneficial effect on human health. One fascinating fact about *Salvia hispanica* is that it produces numerous dry indehiscent fruits, commonly called seeds. Chia, a macro thermal short-day flowering plant, is sown in the late spring season, and it does not show flowering until late summer or fall at high latitudes; therefore, its chances of producing seed are low since grain filling is hampered by frost (Ayerza and Coates, 2005).

Chia seeds could be used as ingredients to enrich foods due to their high nutrients. Many investigations have shown that replacing wheat flour with chia ingredients such as seeds, whole flour, semi-defatted, and low-fat flours affects bakery products' nutritional and functional value. The levels of proteins, lipids, and minerals determined in raw chia flour directly affected the increase of these nutrients. High levels of phytates are found in chia constituents (5.2–6.5 μmol/g d.b.), which affect the bioavailability of Zn and Fe, as predicted by phytate/mineral molar ratios.

Its oil has α-linolenic acid (ALA: 65.4%), linoleic acid (22.5%), unsaturated fatty acids, and less than 12% saturated fatty acids. The seed oil of chia has a low n-6/n-3 ratio; therefore, it could help get the ratio between 5:2 and 8:9, following WHO/FAO (World Health Organization/Food and Agriculture Organization). Chia proteins contain many essential amino acids such as lysine, leucine, isoleucine, and valine. The chia seed proteins have a complete amino acid profile, unlike cereals, which are particularly deficient in lysine. Soluble fiber such as gums, pectins, and mucilages has bioactive effects like enhancing the immune function, lowering cholesterol, and delaying digestion and glucose release from foods, with a consequent decrease in postprandial glycemia.

Many factors cause variations in the concentrations of the active compounds in chia seed; the cultivation area of the plant is one among them. Differences in the environmental conditions with climate changes, type of soil with availabilities of nutrients, time of year of cultivation play crucial roles in the variations. For example, the protein content of chia seeds tends to decrease as the temperature increases. Furthermore, an inverse relationship between altitude and the content of saturated fatty acids had been observed whereby, at low elevation, an increase in fatty acid saturation was noted in areas where the temperature was high. In Argentina, Ayerza demonstrated that temperature largely contributed to the type of fatty acid found in the

DOI: 10.1201/9781003080770-7

oil. They found that, during seed development from April to May, an increase in the environment's temperature decreased the polyunsaturated fatty acid (PUFA) content.

The plant developmental stage is also a factor that may contribute to differences in the chemical compositions of chia seeds. It was observed that the ALA content decreased by 24% from the early stage harvesting to the matured stage of the seed: this concurrently increased linolenic acid (LA) and lignin content.

Different studies have shown the influence of germination on the content of lipids, fiber, protein, ashes, tryptophan, vitamin C, total phenolic, total flavonoid compounds, and protein digestibility antioxidant activity of chia seeds germinated for a few days. The results described that germination for two days increased the protein content of chia seeds by 12% while fiber, tryptophan, total phenolic, and flavonoid contents increased by 47%, 92%, 302%, and 196%, respectively. However, after four days of consecutive germination, Vitamin C was increased to 2.33 mg/100 g. The antioxidant capacity increased approximately 99%, but protein digestibility decreased by 15% on day 4 of germination. Germination can be an excellent method to increase chia seeds' nutritional and nutraceutical potential in designing various functional foods.

We aimed to analyze the physical changes and antioxidant properties of chia seeds roasted under various conditions (160°C–200°C, 5–15 min) and investigate the effects on the quality characteristics of cookies. Weight loss and water-holding capacity rapidly changed after roasting at 180°C. Fatty acid composition showed no significant change, while the antioxidant activity of roasted seeds increased. Cookies were prepared by replacing 3% of the flour with roasted chia seeds (180°C, 0–15 min). Baking gloss, hardness, and brightness were inversely proportional to roasting time.

The processing conditions like hydrolysis time, degree of hydrolysis of the proteins, kind of enzyme, enzyme–substrate ratios, and pretreatment of the protein before hydrolysis may influence the bioactive properties of the protein peptides. Peptide properties can also be influenced by net charge, hydrophobicity, and the size of the peptide, which are factors that affect their absorption across the enterocytes (Udenigwe and Aluko, 2012).

Furthermore, chia seeds' mucilage is linked to starch in bakery products, impeding starch to gelatinize and thus enzymatic vulnerability, and lowering the glycemic index. Moreover, high concentrations of natural antioxidants, such as quercetin and kaempferol, have been found in chia seeds. At the same time, caffeic and chlorogenic acids are present in low concentrations. Chia can be considered a super seed with antioxidative potency and could be used as an antihypertensive substance. Chia has a significant concentration of minerals, but calcium, iron, or zinc's bioavailability depends on the phytate concentration, decreasing during food processing.

Whole chia seeds may be marketed as a food ingredient for products like breakfast cereals up to 11%; ground chia seeds up to 6% in bread; whole chia seeds up to 6% in sterilized ready-to-eat (RTE) meals on cereal/pseudo-cereal grains and pulses. Packaged chia seeds, fruit/nut/seed mixes, baked confectionery goods, chocolates; edible ices; fruit and vegetable products; nonalcoholic beverages, and puddings are also gaining popularity.

The metabolomics profile of four chia seeds early flowering genotype, G3, G8, G17, W13.1, was studied by de Falco et al. (2017) compared to the commercial black and white seeds profile NMR spectroscopy coupled with multivariate data analysis.

Results showed that W 13.1 has the highest content of many bioactive compounds, such as sucrose, raffinose, flavonoids genistein, quercetin, and the caffeoyl derivatives caffeic chlorogenic and rosmarinic acids. The relative content of the identified amino acids was significantly lowest in the G3 and highest in G17, which also showed the highest content of saturated and unsaturated fatty acids. Chia seeds commercialized today have a coat color that ranges from black and black spotted to white. Ayerza (2013a) showed no difference in the chemical composition between two genotypes Tzotzol and Iztac, which produce black-spotted and white seeds, respectively. Chia seeds also increase animal products' x3 fatty acid content like eggs, poultry, and rabbit (Peiretti and Meineri, 2008). Several secondary metabolites belong to the sage seeds, such as flavonoids and their glycosides, polyphenols, mainly composed of caffeic acid building blocks, anthocyanin, and proanthocyanidins. Fiber is a critical component of chia seeds that can be used as a foam stabilizer, suspending agent, and emulsifier for food and pharmaceutical purpose due to its physical properties (Reyes-Caudillo et al., 2008), including water holding capacity and viscosity (Vazquez-Ovando et al., 2009). The chemical composition and each class of compounds in chia seeds vary depending on several factors, including genetic modifications, environmental conditions, and agricultural practices. Chia seeds have a significant role as a functional food and nutritional supplement (Coelho and Salas-Mellado, 2014). Their bioactive compounds' composition and concentration depend on several factors: climatic conditions, geographical origin, and extraction methods (Ayerza and Coates, 2004, 2009a,b, 2011; Capitani et al., 2012; Ixtaina et al., 2011). Seeds comprise total dietary fiber from 47.1% to 59.8% (Weber et al., 1991) and contain up to 40% of oil with high content of unsaturated fatty acids.

Moreover, chia seeds are a good source of proteins (19.3%–26.6%), dietary fiber, vitamins, minerals, and antioxidants (Bushway et al., 1981). It also contains caffeic acid and this phenolic acid (composed of a dihydroxy phenyl group), representing several metabolites' molecular skeleton in the Lamiaceae family. Caffeic acid, also classified as hydroxycinnamic acid, sometimes bounds to quinic acid in different positions to give rise to a class of metabolites called caffeoylquinic acids, of which chlorogenic acid is the most common abundant in chia seeds (Martínez-Cruz and Paredes-López, 2014). Moreover, chia seeds' metabolome presents monomers of caffeic acid building blocks and condensation products such as polymers.

Various monomeric derivatives have been isolated from chia seeds, including caffeic acid and ferulic acid, using ultrahigh performance liquid chromatography (UHPLC) (Martínez-Cruz and Paredes-López, 2014). However, there are no reports from the available literature which show the presence of salvianolic and lithospheric acids in chia seeds. Certain flavonoids and ubiquitous compounds present in plants belong to a polyphenolic subclass and are considered responsible for color, taste, and prevention of oxidative rancidity in fats (Yao et al., 2004). They have widely distributed in chia seeds, and their synthesis increases due to microbial infection (Dixon et al., 1983).

Oil extracted from chia seeds has been used against many physical ailments (Lu and Foo, 2002; Reyes-Caudillo et al., 2008). Chia oil contains a high amount of PUFAs, which range from 25% to 50% (Bushway et al., 1981; Taga et al., 1984). Researchers demonstrated that oil extracted from chia seeds also contains phenolic

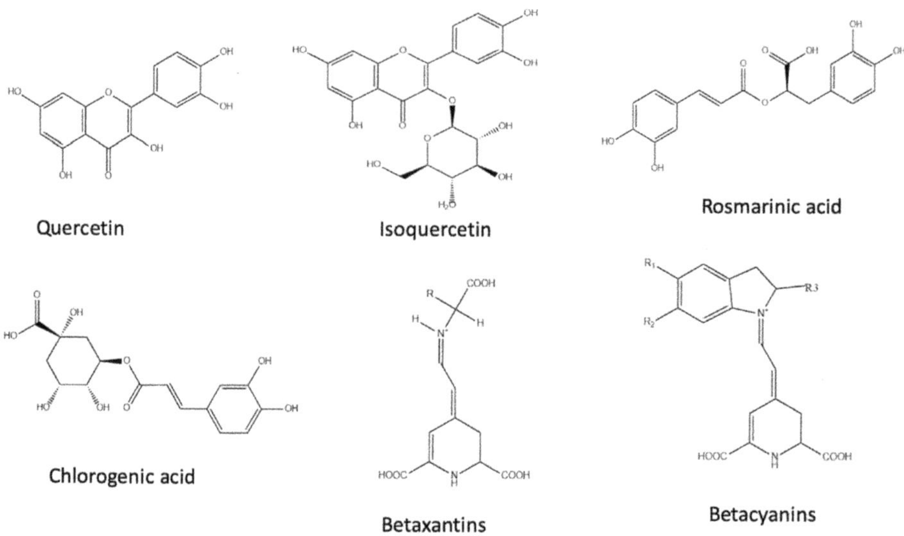

FIGURE 7.1 Chemical structure of the main antioxidant compounds identified in quinoa seeds.

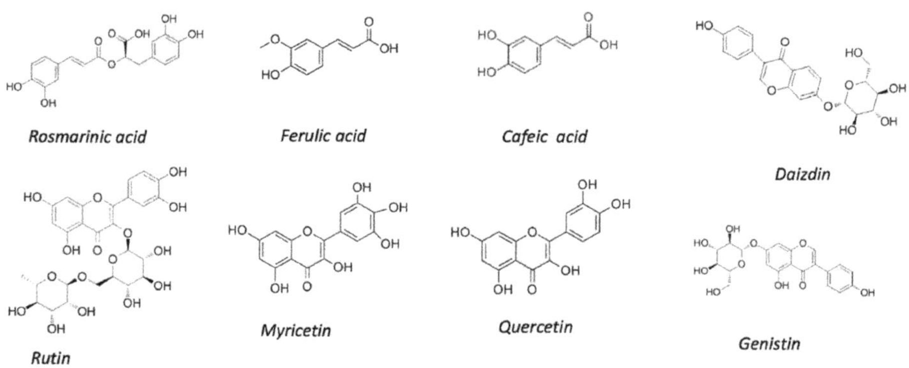

FIGURE 7.2 Chemical structure of the main antioxidant compounds identified in chia seeds.

compounds such as tocopherols, phytosterols, and carotenoids. Their related antioxidant activity plays a significant role in the oil deterioration due to lipid oxidation (Matthaus, 2002; Ixtaina et al., 2011).

It is estimated that consumption of 7.4 g of chia seeds per day may provide 100% of the recommended dose of omega-3 fatty acids, which has been proven helpful in preventing various chronic diseases related to food. Furthermore, chia seeds can be considered a natural source of omega-3, which possess anti-inflammatory and antithrombotic activity (Garg et al., 2006; Geelen et al., 2004; Din et al., 2004; Wall et al., 2010). Another study was done by Amato et al. in 2015, and they found that Italian chia seeds oil is much similar to that which grows in Peru and Australia. However, the oil extracted in Italy was richer in various pigments, including chlorophyll, carotenoids, and a-linolenic acid. The other side shows that these have higher free acidity and peroxide values.

A part of the fiber in chia is located in the outer cells of the fruit. It is partly extruded from the fruit surface upon hydration in a clear mucilaginous capsule that adheres firmly to the fruit itself. Chia seed gum (CSG) is mainly composed of xylose, glucose, arabinose, galactose, glucuronic, and galacturonic acids. However, less information is available about the whole chemical structure of mucilage (Timilsena et al., 2016).

TOTAL POLYPHENOLIC CONTENT AND THEIR ANTIOXIDANT ACTIVITY

Chia seeds contain many natural antioxidants such as tocopherols, phytosterols, carotenoids (Álvarez-Chávez et al., 2008), polyphenolic compounds, which are mainly constructed from the caffeic acid building block and flavonoids, including the flavones myricetin, quercetin, and kaempferol. This class of compounds is the main responsible for the antioxidant activity of chia seeds due to their capability to scavenge free radicals, chelate metal ions, and donate hydrogens. In particular, the B ring of flavones is responsible for ROS and RNS scavenging activity because hydrogen and an electron transfer to hydroxyl, peroxyl, and peroxynitrite radicals, giving a relatively stable flavonoid radical (Cao et al., 1997). Various researchers have confirmed that antioxidant compounds reduce the risk of chronic diseases, including cancer and heart disease. The antioxidant activity of hydrolyzed and nonhydrolyzed extract of chia seeds was also evaluated using b-carotene and linoleic acid (Miller, 1971). Results showed flavones glycosides as the major antioxidant in the nonhydrolyzed extract, followed by chlorogenic and caffeic acid. As mentioned earlier, the place of growth of chia plants affects the chemical composition of chia seeds. da Silva et al. (2017) reported that chia grown in the Rio Grande do Sul showed a higher concentration of lipids, minerals, and antioxidant capacity (478.2 ± 0.02 lmol Trolox equivalence antioxidant capacity [TEAC]/g sample) than chia grown in Mato Grosso (466.3 ± 0.06 lmol TEAC/g sample).

Salvia hispanica L. is a plant known since ancient times whose seeds were used as a primary food in the diet of Mayan and Aztec populations. Chia seeds are considered a good source of nutraceutical components, and several reports have shown their effects on human health due to their chemical composition. They are rich in dietary fiber and PUFAs, especially a-linolenic acid. *S. hispanica* seeds also contain many polyphenols, including caffeic and chlorogenic acids, quercetin, myricetin, and kaempferol, which give high antioxidant activity.

Scientists have conducted various experiments on chia seeds and their products and confirmed their potential health benefits. Chia seeds are found to have hypoglycemic, immune-stimulatory, hypotensive, and antimicrobial effects. The unique ability of chia seeds to absorb enough water and form good gels may be used in food industries as a substitute for emulsifiers and stabilizing agents. In conclusion, chia seeds (*S. hispanica*) are valuable raw materials whose technological and health-promoting properties can be widely used in the food industry.

Soxhlet extraction yields oil with a high absorption capacity, organic molecule absorption, and emulsifying stability. As the main disadvantage, such products containing traces of solvent are unsuitable for applications in the food industry and other branches, producing valuable products for human use. Besides, a slight loss of antioxidant content has been noticed. Modern extraction techniques, such as pressurized liquid extraction based on green chemistry solvents, are being developed as an alternative to traditional methods for oil extraction (Santos et al., 2012). Chia oil obtained by ultrasound-assisted extraction using ethyl acetate as solvent demonstrated high content of FFAs (de Mello et al., 2017; López-Hortas et al., 2018). Supercritical fluid extraction represents a promising alternative extraction method, mainly due to the minor degradation of the bioactive components. CO_2 and n-propane are most frequently used as solvents, preserving oil quality characteristics and selective free lipids from toxic residues. However, n-propane has been demonstrated as a better alternative than CO_2 for oil extraction due to its nonpolarity and consequent high solvent power for lipids. Design of the extraction plant is certainly a complicated procedure, which requires knowledge of phase equilibria and the knowledge of mass transfer rates, determined by the time needed for the extraction. Therefore, it is highly recommended to calculate the extraction process in order to optimize process parameters. Extraction kinetics of supercritical extraction processes have been widely studied to develop optimal extraction models (Bartolomé Ortega et al., 2017; Brunner, 1984; Martínez et al., 2003; Menkiti et al., 2015; Sovová, 2005). Extraction techniques using supercritical fluids have significant advantages over conventional processes due to the lower operating temperatures (suitable for thermolabile fatty acids), absence of organic solvents in the final product (concentrated, high-quality product), no need for further treatment of extract solution (absence of high evaporation temperatures), beneficial environmental impact due to reduced use of solvents in the production process and at industrial scale, batch consistency and compliance with regulatory requirements (quality assurance). Supercritical fluid extraction yields extract free of solvent residues. The obtained products need no further purification in the sense of solvent elimination. Supercritical CO_2, as well as propane, are affordable solvents. Product recovery is completed by a simple pressure reduction method, and compounds in a complex mixture can be selectively separated using the pressure-dependent dissolving power of supercritical fluids. Lesser operating costs are commonly realized since compression energy is more effective than distillation energy. In the present study, *S. hispanica* L. oils have been extracted by subcritical n-propane at two different temperatures, 40°C and 60°C. The operating pressure has been elevated up to 300 bar in order to compare the extraction yield and composition of the extracts with the available literature data (Zanqui et al., 2015) and to verify the aim of obtaining higher extraction yields at higher pressures and temperatures than the ones utilized in the previous studies (Zanqui et al., 2015). Two experiments at the same processing conditions were performed by subjecting the black and white color seeds to the extraction process by the scientists. The influence of extraction conditions and material type on the extraction kinetics has been experimentally determined, and the results were fitted to the mass–transfer model proposed by Brunner (Brunner, 1984). The composition of obtained oils was determined via gas chromatography. The concentration of critical compounds omega-3and omega-6 was compared in the extracts obtained by subcritical extraction with n-propane and extracts obtained with Soxhlet and ultrasonic extraction using n-hexane.

Germination: Antioxidant activity and phenolic content are greatly affected by domestic processing – germination of quinoa results in increased values of oleic acid. However, linoleic acid decreased in NL (nonpolar lipids), GL, and PL. The ratio of saturated, monounsaturated, and PUFAs of NL and PL approached 3: 4: 3. After 72 hours of germination, the ratio of Omega3/6 became 0.25 in GL (glycolipids) (Park and Naofumi, 2004). The antinutrients such as tannin and phytate contents could not be detected after steeping and germination in a study conducted by Kanensi et al. in 2011. Germination resulted in a twofold increase in antioxidant activity after three days of germination. The amounts of phenolic acids and flavonoids increased 8.57-fold and 4.4-fold, respectively (Carciochi et al., 2013). Germination and subsequent oven-drying are excellent processes to improve quinoa seed's phenolic content and antioxidant activity and can be used to form functional foods. The germinated products contain essential fatty acids that play a vital health beneficial role in the development of the brain, insulin sensitivity, prostaglandin metabolism. When fermentation was carried out in the natural environment by the microorganisms present in the seeds or by inoculation with two *Saccharomyces cerevisiae* strains used for baking and brewing, there was decreased ascorbic acid and tocopherol content, and the phenolic compounds and antioxidant capacity were improved (Carciochi et al., 2016). Malting with a moderate thermal treatment is an effective process to enhance antioxidants in quinoa grains for the production of gluten-free foods and beverages (Carciochi et al., 2016).

Dehydration: Dehydration of quinoa between 70°C and 80°C brings an increase in vitamin E content, and the antioxidant capacity was also found to be increased on dehydration at 40°C, 50°C, and 80°C due to temperature/drying time equivalent processes. The dehydration process in quinoa resulted in reductions of 10.1% in proteins, 11.9% in fat, and 26.8% in both fiber and ash content (Miranda et al., 2010). The heat application to quinoa has shown a reduction of antinutritional factors in *Chenopodium quinoa* seeds (Silva et al., 2015).

Heat processing: This is required for the complete digestion of food proteins. Heat treatments at different temperatures significantly affect the structure of the protein. Extrusion processing is mainly used to make extruded RTE breakfast cereals from quinoa fortified with fruit concentrates. The extrudates contain higher phenolic values, which may be due to the formation of Maillard products at higher barrel temperatures and maximum anthocyanins content of 9.64 mg/kg d.m at 142°C (Chandran, 2015). Extrusion results in the inactivation of antinutrients, destruction of aflatoxins, and increasing the digestibility of fiber (Saalia and Phillips, 2011). Extrusion results in the transformation of insoluble dietary fiber to a soluble dietary form. This results in the formation of resistant starch and enzyme-resistant glucans through the process of transglycosylation (Repo-Carrasco-Valencia and Serna, 2009). High extrusion temperatures in the extrudates of quinoa resulted in the inactivation of antinutrients. Also, oxidation of unsaturated fatty acids results in decreased content of unsaturated fatty acids due to high extrusion temperatures (Chandran, 2015).

Roasted quinoa seeds flour at 178°C for 15, 30 and 45 minutes resulted in an increased final viscosity of cakes, weakening of starch–protein interactions, and swelling of the starch granules, leading to granule rupture and decreased geometric mean diameters with elevated roasting temperatures (Rothschild et al., 2014).

Baking: Baking red and yellow quinoa seeds resulted in a beneficial increase in total phenolic content and antioxidant activity. As discussed earlier, this increase in antioxidant activity happened due to the Maillard reaction products produced due to thermal processing (Brend et al., 2012).

High pressure: High temperature processed quinoa products increased iron solubility two to four times after soaking and germination, 3–5 times after fermentation, and 5–8 times after the germinated flour ferment. 5–8 times in magnesium content has been improved after cooking and baking, and copper content was reduced by 28% after processing (Ruiz and Opazo-Navarrete, 2016).

Quinoa is mainly utilized in meat products such as burgers, meatballs, nuggets, bolognas, pâté, and dry-cured sausages. It is used as a functional ingredient due to its high protein and carbohydrate content, or it may be used as a fat replacer in products due to its behavior as a fat-like raw material. However, although these have been the primary purpose, several authors have reported that their addition helped control the development of rancidity due to lipid oxidation in the meat product. Özer and Seçen added quinoa flour (up to 10%; in substitution of breadcrumbs) to beef burgers with the corresponding improvement in burger quality and cooking properties.

Additionally, they also found that quinoa flour inhibited lipid oxidation during frozen storage. The antioxidant effect of quinoa flour was identified in raw beef burgers at all usage rates (3%, 5%, 7%, and 10%) during −18°C storage for 90 days. These antioxidant properties of quinoa flour were also observed when these burgers were cooked, attributing this antioxidant effect to the phenolic and flavonoid content in quinoa as a source of free radical scavenging agents. Fernández-López et al. investigated the application of black quinoa seeds (as whole seeds or as their fiber-rich fraction obtained as a coproduct from the quinoa wet-milling process) in bologna-type sausages (up to 3%; in substitution of potato starch). These authors reported that it was a feasible strategy for reformulating cooked sausages and maybe a good choice not only for enhancing the nutritional composition of the bolognas but also for their effect on the technological properties, such as enhancing emulsion stability to decrease lipid oxidation. In addition, Lin et al. reported that the compounds having antioxidant properties in quinoa seeds are located in the inner of the grain, and only a reduced amount has been identified in bran. The antioxidant effect of black quinoa seeds in bolognas was also found to be increased with their refrigerated storage.

Many researchers have attributed the antioxidant activity of quinoa seeds is only due to their hydrophilic phytochemicals, mainly phenolics. However, the contribution of lipophilic compounds (tocopherols and carotenoids) must not be underestimated. About the antioxidant properties of quinoa grains (black, white, and colored varieties) attributed to their phenolic compounds, they were assessed using different methods, being the most usual DPPH (0.1–9.7 mg TE/g), ABTS (3.88–7.76 mg TE/g), ferric ion reducing antioxidant power (FRAP) (0.7–9 mg TE/g), and ferrous ion chelating (FIC) (0.59–0.97 μg EDTA/g) assays. The results showed a good correlation with phenols and flavonoids content. For all assays, red and black quinoa seeds showed better antioxidant activities than white varieties.

Variation in the antioxidant capacity of chia and quinoa may be expected, as many factors such as genetics, agrotechnical processes, and environmental conditions can influence the presence of various phenolic compounds. Several antioxidant capacity assays have been applied by many scientists mainly to evaluate the chemical mechanism involved in the antioxidative action. Depending upon the reactions involved, these assays can be classified into two types: hydrogen atom transfer (oxygen radical absorbance capacity assay and total radical trapping antioxidant parameter, and assays based on electron transfer (TEAC assay or ABTS assay, FRAP and the DPPH-free radical method). In addition, other methods are used to evaluate their chelating activity on specific pro-oxidants, such as the method to measure the FIC activity. We can say that the FRAP assay measures the ability of quinoa and chia seeds to reduce ferric ion, DPPH, and ABTs assays measure the radical quencher ability, and the FIC assay the ability to quench iron.

The antioxidant effect of quinoa grains is attributed to polyphenols, natural organic chemicals with phenol as structural units. The TPC reported in quinoa grains by scientists ranged between 0.4 and 10.9 mg. Darker varieties of quinoa seeds, such as red and black, showed higher total phenolic contents than white varieties. The color of quinoa grains, phenolic profiles, and antioxidant activity decide the variable TPC values. Several authors have recently reported that the malting process increases the number of phenolic compounds. In quinoa flour; an up to 48% increase in TPC compared to the initial content before malting. Scientists also reported that the increase in TPC was higher in flour from colored quinoa seeds (red and black) than white ones. Ballester-Sánchez et al. determined the polyphenol fractions, extractable and hydrolyzable present in red quinoa seeds, and the fiber-rich fractions obtained by the dry and wet-milling process. The values reported for the extractable fraction were 4.8 mg GAE/g for the whole seeds and 3.7 mg GAE/g and 6.5 mg GAE/g for the fractions from wet and dry milling, respectively. The results may conclude that the wet-milling fiber portion shows lower values in the extractable polyphenol fraction than the whole seeds, whereas they were the same in the case of the fiber fraction from dry-milling.

BIBLIOGRAPHY

Álvarez-Chávez, L. M., Valdivia-López, M. D. L. A., Aburto-Juarez, M. D. L., and Tecante, A. (2008). Chemical characterization of the lipid fraction of Mexican chia seed (Salvia hispanica L.). *Int J Food Prop* 11:687–697.

Ayerza, R. (2013a). Seed composition of two chia (Salvia his-panica L.) genotypes which differ in seed color Emir. *J Food Agric* 25:495–500.

Ayerza, R. and Coates, W. (2004). Protein and oil content, peroxide index and fatty acid composition of chia (Salvia hispanica L.) grown in six tropical and subtropical ecosystems of South America. *Trop Sci* 44(3):131–135.

Ayerza, R. and Coates, W. (2005). Effect of ground chia seed and chia oil on plasma total cholesterol, LDL, HDL, triglyceride content, and fatty acid composition when fed to rats. *Nutr Res* 11:995–1003.

Ayerza, R. and Coates, W. (2009a). Some quality components of four chia (Salvia hispanica L.) genotypes grown under tropical coastal desert ecosystem conditions. *Asian J Plant Sci* 8(4):301–307.

Ayerza, R. and Coates, W. (2009b). Influence of environment on growing period and yield, protein, oil and linolenic content of three chia (Salvia hispanica L.) selections. *Ind Crop Prod* 30:321–324.

Ayerza, R. and Coates, W. (2011). Protein content, oil content and fatty acid profiles as potential criteria to determine the origin of commercially grown chia (Salvia hispanica L.). *Ind Crop Prod* 34:1366–1371.

Bartolomé Ortega, A. B., Calvo Garcia, A., Szekely, E., Škerget, M., and Knez, Ž. (2017). Supercritical fluid extraction from Saw Palmetto berries at a pressure range between 300 bar and 450 bar. *J Supercrit Fluids* 120:132–139.

Brend, Y., Galili, L., Badani, H., Hovav, R., and Galili, S. (2012). Total phenolic content and antioxidant activity of red and yellow quinoa (Chenopodium quinoa Wild) seeds as affected by baking and cooking conditions. *Food Nutr Sci* 3:1150–1155.

Brunner, G. (1984). Mass transfer from solid material in gas extraction, Berichte Bunsenges. *Für Phys Chem* 88:887–891.

Bushway, A. A., Belya, P. R., and Bushway, R. J. (1981). Chia seed as a source of oil, polysaccharide, and protein. *J Food Sci* 46:1349e1356.

Cao, G., Sofic, E., and Prior ,R. L. (1997). Antioxidant and prooxidant behavior of flavonoids: Structure-activity relationships. *Free Radic Biol Med* 22:749–760.

Capitani, M. I., Spotorno, V., Nolasco, S. N., and Tomás, M. C. (2012). Physicochemical and functional characterization of by-products from chia (*Salvia hispanica* L.) seeds of Argentina. *LWT—Food Sci Technol* 45:94–102.

Carciochi, R. A., Dimitrov, K., and Galván D´Alessandro, L. (2013). Effect of malting conditions on phenolic content, Maillard reaction products formation, and antioxidant activity of quinoa seeds. *J Food Sci Technol*, 1–8.

Carciochi, R. A., Galván-D'Alessandro, L., and Vandendriessche, P. (2016). Effect of germination and fermentation process on the antioxidant compounds of quinoa seeds. *Plant Foods Human Nutr* 71(4):361–367.

Chandran, S. (2015). Effect of extrusion on physico-chemical properties of quinoa-cassava extrudates fortified with cranberry concentrate. Thesis. Graduate School-New Brunswick Rutgers, The State University of New Jersey, 45–61.

Coelho, M. S. and Salas-Mellado, M. M. (2014). Chemical characterization of CHIA (Salvia hispanica L.) for use in food products. *J Food Nutr Res* 2(5):263–269.

da Silva, B. P., Anunciação, P. C., Matyelka, J. C. da. S., Della Lucia, C. M., Martino, H. S. D., and Pinheiro-Sant'Ana, H. M. (2017). Chemical composition of Brazilian chia seeds grown in different places. *Food Chem* 221:1709–1716.

de Falco, B., Incerti, G., Bochicchio, R., Phillips, T. D., Amato, M., and Lanzotti, V. (2017). Metabolomic analysis of Salvia his-panica seeds using NMR spectroscopy and multivariate data analysis. *Ind Crop Prod* 99:86–96.

De Mello, B. T. F., Dos Santos Garcia, V. A., and Da Silva, C. (2017). Ultrasound-assisted extraction of oil from chia (Salvia hispânica L.) seeds: Optimization extraction and fatty acid profile. *J Food Process Eng* 40:e12298.

Din, J. N., Newby, D. E., and Flapan, A. D. (2004). Omega 3 fatty acids and cardiovascular disease—fishing for a natural treatment. *Br Med J* 328:30–35

Dixon, R. A., Dey, P. M., and Lamb, C. J. (1983). Phytoalexins: Enzymology and molecular biology. *Adv Enzymol Relat Areas Mol Biol* 55:1–136.

Dweck, A. C. (2005). The folklore cosmetic use of various salvia spices. In: *Sage the Genus Salvia*. S. E. Kitzios (Ed.). Handbook Academic Publishers, Amsterdam, 1–25.

Garg, M. L., Wood, L. G., Singh, H., and Moughan, P. J. (2006). Means of delivering recommended levels of long chain n-3polyunsaturated fatty acids in human diets. *J Food Sci* 71:66–71.

Geelen, A., Brouwer, I. A., Zock, P. L., and Katan, M. B. (2004). Antiarrhythmic effects of n-3 fatty acids: Evidence from human studies. *Curr Opin Lipidol* 15:25–30.

Ixtaina, V. Y., Martínez, M. L., Spotorno, V., Mateo, C. M., Maestri, D. M., Diehl, B. W. K., and Tomás, M. C. (2011). Characterization of chia seed oils obtained by pressing and solvent extraction. *J Food Compos Anal* 24:166–174.

López-Hortas, L., Pérez-Larrán, P., González-Muñoz, M. J., and Falqué, E, and Domínguez, H. (2018). Recent developments on the extraction and application of ursolic acid. A review. *Food Res. Int.* 103:130–149.

Lu, Y., and Foo, L. Y. (2002). Polyphenolics of Salvia—A review. *Phytochemistry* 59:117–140.

Martínez, J., Monteiro, A. R., Rosa, P. T. V., Marques, M. O. M., and Meireles, M. A. A. (2003). Multicomponent model to describe extraction of ginger oleoresin with supercritical carbon dioxide. *Ind Eng Chem Res* 42:1057–1063.

Martínez-Cruz, O. and Paredes-López, O. (2014). Phytochemical profile and nutraceutical potential of chia seeds (*Salvia hispanica* L.) by ultra-high performance liquid chromatography. *J Chromatogr A* 1346:43–48.

Matthaus, B. (2002). Antioxidant activity of extracts obtained from residues of different oilseeds. *J Agric Food Chem* 50:3444–3452.

Menkiti, M. C., Agu, C. M., and Udeigwe, T. K. (2015). Extraction of oil from *Terminalia catappa* L.: Process parameter impacts, kinetics, and thermodynamics. *Ind Crops Prod* 77:713–723.

Miller, H. E. (1971). A simplified method for the evaluation ofantioxidants. *J Am Oil Chem Soc* 48:91–105.

Miranda, M., Vega-Gálvez, A., López, J., Parada, G., Sanders, M., and Aranda, M. (2010). Impact of air-drying temperature on nutritional properties, total phenolic content and antioxidant capacity of quinoa seeds (Chenopodium quinoa Willd.). *Ind Crops Product* 32:258–263.

Miranda, M., Vega-Gálvez, A., Martínez, E., López, J., Rodriquez, M. J., Henriquez, K., and Fuentes, F. (2012). Genetic diversity and comparison of physiochemical and nutritional characteristics of six quinoa (Chenopodium quinoa Willd) genotypes cultivated in Chile. *Ciênc Tecnol Aliment Campinas.* 32(4):835–843.

Park, S. H. and Naofumi, M. (2004). Changes of bound lipids and composition of fatty acids in germination of quinoa seeds. *Food Sci Technol* 10(3):303–306.

Peiretti, P. G. and Meineri, G. (2008). Effects on growth performance, carcass characteristics, and the fat and meat fatty acid profile of rabbits fed diets with Chia (Salvia hispanica L.) seed supplements. *Meat Sci* 80:1161–1121.

Repo-Carrasco-Valencia, R. and Serna, L. A. (2009). Quinoa (Chenopodium quinoa, Willd.) as a source of dietary fiber and other functional components. *Food Sci Technol (Campinas)* 31(1):225–230.

Reyes-Caudillo, E., Tecante, A., and Valdivia-Lopez, M. A. (2008). Dietary fibre content and antioxidant activity of phenolic compounds present in Mexican chia (Salvia hispanica L.) seeds. *Food Chem* 107(2):656–663.

Rothschild, J., Hoddy, K. K., Jambazian, P., and Varady, K. A. (2014). Time-restricted feeding and risk of metabolic disease: A review of human and animal studies. *Nutr Rev* 72:308–318.

Ruiz, G. A. and Opazo-Navarrete, M. (2016). Exploring novel food proteins and processing technologies: A case study on quinoa protein and high pressure-high temperature processing. Thesis.

Saalia, F. and Phillips, R. D. (2011). Degradation of aflatoxins by extrusion cooking: Effects on nutritional quality of extrudates. *LWT-Food Sci Technol* 44(6):1496–1501.

Santos, G. M., Alexandre, A., Southon, J. R., Treseder, K. K., Corbineau, R., and Reyerson, P. E. (2012). Possible source of ancient carbon in phytolith concentrates from harvested grasses. *Biogeosciences* 9:1873–1884.

Silva, J. A., Pompeu, G., Olavo, C., Gonçalves, D. B., and Spehar, C. R. (2015). The importance of heat against antinutritional factors from Chenopodium quinoa seeds. *Food Sci Technol* 35(1):74–82.

Sovová, H. (2005). Mathematical model for supercritical fluid extraction of natural products and extraction curve evaluation. *J Supercrit Fluids* 33:35–52.

Taga, M. S., Miller, E. E., and Pratt, D. E. (1984). Chia seeds as a source of natural lipid antioxidants. *J Am Oil Chem Soc* 61:928–932.

Timilsena, Y. P., Adhikari, R., Kasapis, S., and Adhikari, B. (2016). Molecular and functional characteristics of purified gum from Australian chia seeds. *Carbohydr Polym* 136:128–136.

Udenigwe, C. C. and Aluko, R. E. (2012). Food protein-derived bioactive peptides: Production, processing, and potential health benefits. *J Food Sci* 77(1):R11–R24.

Vazquez-Ovando, A., Rosado-Rubio, G., Chel-Guerrero, L., & Betancur-Ancona, D. (2009). Physicochemical properties of a fibrous fraction from chia (*Salvia hispanica* L). *LWT Food Sci Technol* 42:168–173.

Wall, R., Ross, R. P., Fitzgerald, G. F., and Stanton, C. (2010). Fatty acids from fish: The anti-inflammatory potential of long-chainomega-3 fatty acids. *Nutr Rev* 68:280–289.

Weber, C. W., Gentry, H. S., Kohlhepp, E. A., and McCrohan, P. R. (1991). The nutritional and chemical evaluation of chia seeds. *Ecol Food Nutr* 26:119–125.

Yao, L. H., Jiang, Y. M., Shi, J., Tomas-Barberan, F. A., Datta, N., Sin-ganusong, R., and Chen, S. S. (2004). Flavonoids in food and their health benefits. *Plant Food Hum Nutr* 59:113–122.

Zanqui, A. B., de Morais, D. R., da Silva, C. M., Santos, J. M., Chiavelli, L. U. R., Bittencourt, P. R. S. et al. (2015). Subcritical extraction of salvia hispanica L. oil with N-propane: Composition, purity and oxidation stability as compared to the oils obtained by conventional solvent extraction methods. *J Braz Chem Soc* 26:282–289.

8 Quinoa Products

Quinoa (*Chenopodium quinoa*) is a species of goosefoot (Chenopodium), a grain crop grown primarily for its edible seeds. It is a staple food of ancient civilizations and got originated in the Andean region of South America. It is a tiny seed that looks like a cross between sesame seeds and millets. Quinoa (the name is derived from the Spanish spelling of the Quechua name kinwa or occasionally 'qin wah'. All crops, referred to as pseudocereals, resemble in function and composition those of the true cereals. In quinoa seeds, the embryo or germ, which is circular, surrounds the starch-rich perisperm and together with the seed coat represents the bran fraction which is relatively rich in fat and protein.

Quinoa may benefit high-risk group consumers, such as children, the elderly, high-performance sportspeople, individuals with lactose intolerance, women prone to osteoporosis, people with anemia, diabetes, dyslipidemia, obesity, and celiac disease due to its properties including a high nutritional value, therapeutic features, and gluten-free content (Table 8.1). These features are considered linked with the fiber, minerals, vitamins, fatty acids, antioxidants, and especially phytochemicals in quinoa. They provide quinoa a significant advantage over other crops in terms of human nutrition and health maintenance.

Quinoa's tendency to produce high protein grains under ecologically extreme conditions makes it necessary to diversify agriculture in high-altitude regions of the Himalayas and North Indian Plains. Quinoa is a treasure trove of nutrients. The quinoa seed protein is rich in essential amino acids (EAA), particularly methionine, threonine, and lysine, limiting amino acids in most cereal grains. Unlike wheat, rice, and corn, which are low in lysine, quinoa contains a balanced set of EAA such as methionine, cysteine, and lysine, making quinoa an excellent complement to legumes that are limiting in these amino acids. Grains of quinoa contain large amounts of minerals like calcium, iron, zinc, and copper. Quinoa contains 4.4%–8.8% crude fat with the essential fatty acids linoleic and linolenic acid accounting for 55%–63% of the total fatty acids and has a lipid-lowering effect. The main flavonoids in quinoa are kaempferol and quercetin, and both are solid antioxidants and free-radical scavengers. A pseudocereal contains gluten-free high-quality protein to play an essential role in the diet of people who have celiac disease. Celiac disease is considered one of the most common lifelong disorders worldwide, with an estimated mean prevalence of 1% of the general population. The only acceptable treatment for celiac disease is the strict lifelong elimination of gluten from the diet.

Chenopodium is an under-exploited vegetable that has high functional potential apart from essential nutritional benefits. The plant is used in the diet to provide minerals, fiber, vitamins, and essential fatty acids and enhance the sensory and functional value of the food (Poonia and Upadhayay, 2015). The tender shoots are eaten raw in a salad or curd; they are also cooked as a vegetable curry; the cooked shoots can also be mixed with yogurt/curd and eaten raw. The dried part is

DOI: 10.1201/9781003080770-8

TABLE 8.1
Products from Quinoa

Product	Ingredients Used: Control (100% Refined Wheat Flour)	Test Sample	Method
Cookies	Refined flour (100 g) Powdered Sugar (50 g) Fat (58 g) Milk (11 mL) Baking powder (2 g)	Quinoa flour (10 g) Rice flour (45 g) Oats flour (45 g) Powdered Sugar (50 g) Fat (Dalda) (58 g) Milk (11 mL) Baking powder (2 g)	(1) Fat was rubbed on a clean surface. (2) Flours were sifted and baking powder was added gradually. Sugar was added in it. (3) Smooth dough was made by using milk and rolled to ¼ inch thickness. (4) Round shapes were cut and baked at 150° C for 20 minutes.
Cakes	Refined flour (100 g) Powdered Sugar (100 g) Butter (50 g) Eggs (80 g) Baking powder (2 g) Vanilla essence (4 mL)	Quinoa flour (10 g) Rice flour (45 g) Oats flour (45 g) Powdered Sugar (100 g) Fat (Butter) (50 g) Eggs (80 g) Baking powder (2 g) Vanilla essence (4 mL)	(1) Flours and baking powder were sifted twice. (2) Fat and sugar were creamed together till light and fluffy. (3) Eggs were beaten along with vanilla essence. (4) Beaten eggs were added to the creamy mixture little by little mixing continuously. (5) Flour was folded gently using cut-and-fold method. (6) Milk was added to bring the mixture to dropping consistency. (7). Mixture was poured in a greased cake tin and was appropriately leveled. (8) Cake was baked at 180°C for 20 minutes.
Muffins	Refined flour (100 g) Powdered Sugar (100 g) Refined oil (42 g) Butter (33 g) Eggs (167 g) Baking powder (2 g) Vanilla essence (4 mL)	Quinoa flour (10 g) Rice flour (45 g) Oats flour (45 g) Powdered Sugar (100 g) Refined oil (42 g) Butter (33 g) Eggs (167 g) Baking powder (2 g) Vanilla essence (4 mL)	(1) Flours with baking powder were sifted twice. (2) Eggs were beaten in a bowl. (3) Vanilla essence and sugar were added and mixed till the contents became very stiff. (4) Melted butter was added and mixed well. (5) Enameled bowl containing beaten eggs was taken out from hot water. (6) Flour was added gradually and gently mixed with other ingredients. (7) Mixture was poured into prepared muffin tray. (8) Muffins were baked at 200°C for 20 minutes.
Pies	Refined flour (100 g) Butter (67 g) Powdered Sugar (33 g) Baking Powder (3 g) For filling: Sponge cake gluten free (20 g) Apple (chopped) (20 g) Sugar (10 g) Cinnamon powder (10 g) Raisins (5 g)	Quinoa flour (10 g) Rice flour (45 g) Oats flour (45 g) Butter (67 g) Powdered Sugar (33 g) Baking Powder (3 g) For filling: Sponge cake (gluten-free) (20 g) Apple (chopped) (20 g) Sugar (10 g) Cinnamon powder (10 g) Raisins (5 g)	(1) Butter and sugar were creamed with hands and palms on flat surface. (2) Flours were added and mixed it with hands by rubbing with palm. (3) Flattened with rolling pin to ¼ inch thickness. (4) Rolled dough was placed on the apple pie molds. (5) Extra edges were cut using knife. (6) Shaped dough was pricked with fork. (7) All the ingredients were mixed together for filling. (8) Small amount of water was taken in a pan and cooked the mixture for 2–3 minutes. (9) The mixture was placed in pie tray and strips were placed on top. (10) Pies were baked at 200°C for 20 minutes.

(Continued)

TABLE 8.1 (*Continued*)
Products from Quinoa

Product	Ingredients Used: Control (100% Refined Wheat Flour)	Ingredients Used: Test Sample	Method
Tarts	Refined flour (100 g) Butter (67 g) Powdered Sugar (35 g) Baking powder (2.5 g) For filling: Whipped cream (20 g) Chocolate sauce (20 g) Mango (10 g) Kiwi (10 g)	Quinoa flour (10 g) Rice flour (45 g) Oats flour (45 g) Butter (67 g) Powdered Sugar (35 g) Baking powder (2.5 g) For filling: Whipped cream (20 g) Chocolate sauce (20 g) Mango (10 g) Kiwi (10 g)	(1) Fat and sugar were creamed together. (2) Flours and baking powder were mixed with fingers. (3) Balls were made and kept for rest for 10–15 minutes. (4) Balls were flattened with rolling pin and the shapes were cut with doughnut cutter. (5) Flattened balls were placed in tart mold and pricked with fork. (6) Extra batter was trimmed from sides of molds. (7) Tarts were baked at 180°C for 20 minutes.

Source: Natural Science Foundation https://journals.ansfoundation.org/index.php/jans/article/download/1552/1487/2934

stored for future use. The leaves are rich in potassium and vitamin C. Chemically, leaves are found to contain various components such as moisture (89.66%), protein (3.6%), fat (0.5%), other carbohydrates (2.8%), minerals (2.7 g), calcium (14 g), phosphorus (7 g), iron(4.3 g), thiamine (0.02 mg), niacin (0.7 mg), vitamin C (35 mg), carotene (1.471 μg), along with traces of iodine, fluorine, and vitamin K. (Pande et al., 2009).

With increased production and consumption of quinoa, new industrialized quinoa products were produced and manufactured. Quinoa flour is among the major products that are developed from quinoa seeds. Quinoa flour is versatile because it is used in almost all bakery products such as bread, pasta, sponge cakes, or biscuits). Quinoa flour can also be used to produce quinoa noodles specifically. The utilization of quinoa flour for the production of noodles offers an alternative for celiac disease or gluten sensitivity and creates a product with different organoleptic characteristics than regular noodles. Studies are yet to be expected to define recommended quinoa cultivars more appropriate for the noodles and pasta industry.

Furthermore, quinoa flakes can be considered one of the new quinoa products produced by drying and pressing processes. It is assumed that the characteristics of the flakes will depend on the variety of quinoa used, as the plasticity characteristics of quinoa will vary with different quinoas. Quinoa flakes are used in juices, soups, pies, or cakes as they require less cooking time than other grains. Many other options create expanded quinoa products (or pisan Kalla) made from the pearled grain. Quinoa-based extruded products are also developed during the past years as new quinoa food products. The extrusion processes involve high pressure and temperatures, as well as shearing over short periods. Different textures are produced because of this process as it restructures the starch and protein content of quinoa.

The physicochemical reactions happening during extrusion processing of quinoa involve the following:

a. gelatinization and dextrinization of starch, texturing of protein, and denaturation of the vitamins present;
b. plasticizing and melting of the food, and
c. expansion by using flash evaporators for removal of moisture.

Pearled quinoa is fed into the extruder, undergoing a machine and thermal transition to form the semi-solid dough. This dough is then extruded through the machine and sheared at the outlet with a rotary cutter to obtain the final product. There is no nutritional degradation of quinoa in this process, probably due to shorter processing times.

QUINOA PRODUCTS

Day by day, quinoa products have been diversified in international markets. Citizens now welcome new products of quinoa like sprouts, noodles, and cakes in developed countries.

At present, in addition to the basic and primary products of quinoa grain and flour, various other food products, such as noodles, flakes, steamed bread, flavored cakes, and biscuits, can also be found in the domestic market (Li et al., 2018; Liu et al., 2018). Quinoa can also be used for yogurt, yellow wine, and liquor production (Li et al., 2018).

COOKIES

In terms of nutritional composition, quinoa is excellent as compared to common cereals. Cookies have become one of the most desirable snacks nowadays. Demir and Kilinç (2017) used quinoa flour instead of wheat flour in cookies. They used different proportions of quinoa flour in cookie formulation (0%, 10%, 20%, 30%, 40%, and 50%) and analyzed its effects on cookies' physical, chemical, nutritional, and sensory properties. The addition of quinoa flour led to a slight increase in the product thickness. In contrast, the diameter decreases with the increase in quinoa flour in cookie formulation (a significant decrease was observed above 20% addition).

Quinoa flour increased the crude protein, ash, crude fat, and total phenolic content (TPC) of cookie samples. Also, an increase in phytic acid was observed in cookies having quinoa flour. An increase in quinoa flour addition leads to an increase in minerals like potassium (K), magnesium (Mg), calcium (Ca), iron (Fe), and zinc (Zn) contents of the cookies.

Moreover, quinoa flour cookies have overall acceptability in terms of color, taste, crispness except for odor scores. They concluded that cookies with quinoa flour were satisfactorily improved in terms of chemical, nutritional and sensory properties nutritional properties.

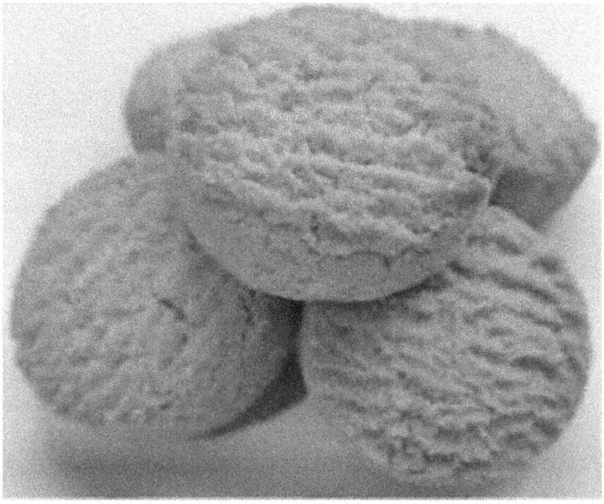

FIGURE 8.1 Quinoa cookies.

GLUTEN-FREE BAKERY PRODUCTS

Nowadays, food manufacturers use whole grains, including corn, rice, sorghum, buckwheat, amaranth, and quinoa to produce gluten-free foods. Most of these are excellent sources of fiber, iron, and vitamin B sources.

Shehry (2016) substituted corn flour with quinoa flour to produce gluten-free bakery products such as pan bread or biscuits in autism disease and celiac cases nutrition. They used quinoa flour as a substitute at 25%, 50%, and 75% for corn flour. They observed that due to high protein, ash, fiber, fat, and mineral content in quinoa flour, corn flour led to an increase in protein, ash, fiber, and fat, and improved the nutritional characteristics of the final product.

However, a continuous increase in quinoa flour showed decreased physical and sensory characteristics in pan bread and biscuits. In total, 25% and 50% addition of quinoa flour showed acceptable sensory and physical properties in both biscuits and panned bread with a significant improvement in the nutritional qualities.

QUINOA FLAKES

Flake is a small, flat, fragile piece of something, typically one which has been peeled off or broken away from a more significant piece. Quinoa is considered a sacred plant and has an exceptional nutritional balance

Quinoa can be used as a good source of a gluten-free diet for people who cannot digest gluten in their intestines. It is also considered as a complete food, quinoa flakes and corn flakes which provides a good amount of fat, protein, carbohydrates, and energy along with saturated, unsaturated fatty acids (MUFA, PUFA) and ash (Prince et al., 2018)

Quinoa flakes are rich in many minerals (Fe, Zn, Ca, Mg, Na, K, P, Cu, and Mn). Quinoa flakes and corn flakes also provide a significant amount of vitamin B1, B2, B3

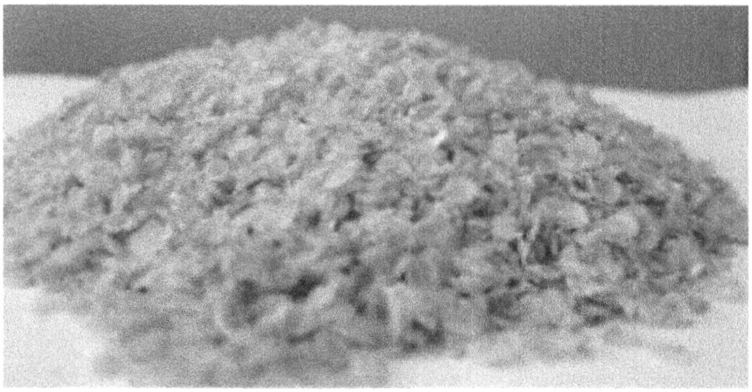

FIGURE 8.2 Quinoa flakes.

and C which were 0.34, 0.40, 1.11, 5.02 (mg/100 g) and 0.89, 1.07, 3.57, 10.21(mg/100 g), respectively.

Both are considered rich sources of macronutrients and micronutrients. So as a concluding remark, quinoa flakes and corn flakes both are good for cardiovascular health, brain health, and the human body.

QUINOA PROTEIN

The protein of quinoa in quantity and quality is superior to other cereal grains; it also has a gluten-free property and high digestibility.

Quinoa has high total protein content (12.9%–16.5%), globulin and albumin are major storage proteins with little to no prolamins. Quinoa exhibits remarkable nutritional properties, not just because of its high protein content (15%) but also from its excellent amino acid balance. Quinoa protein is rich in amino acids like lysine and methionine that are deficient in cereal proteins.

The grain is used to make quinoa flour, soup, breakfast cereals, and alcohol, while the flour is mainly utilized in making biscuits, bread, and processed food. Quinoa starch has tiny grains, and high viscosity can be exploited for various industrial applications. It has also been found to contain minor compounds like phytosterols and

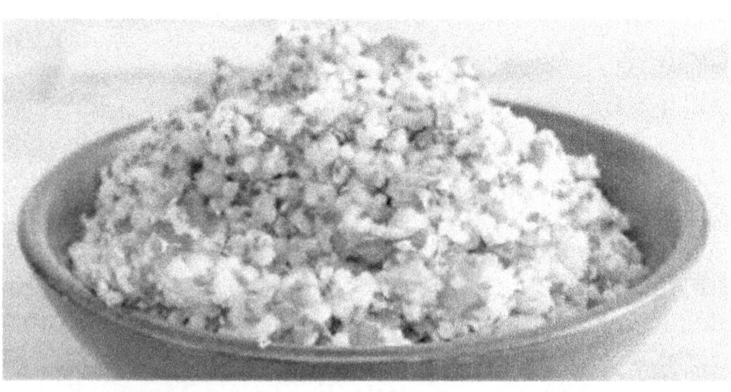

FIGURE 8.3 Quinoa protein.

flavonoids with possible nutraceutical benefits. Quinoa starch has functional (technological) properties like solubility, good water-holding capacity, gelation, emulsifying, and foaming capacity, allowing diversified uses. Mainly, it has been considered an oil crop, with an exciting proportion of omega-6 and unique vitamin-E content. Quinoa starch has physico-chemical properties (such as viscosity and freeze stability), giving it functional properties with novel uses. Quinoa has a high nutritional value and has recently been used as a novel functional food because of all these properties, investigated by Sharma et al. (2015).

QUINOA PORRIDGE

Quinoa porridge is prepared as a highly nutritional diet in India. Quinoa flakes are boiled in milk or water with lots of green vegetables and peanuts. It makes it a complete source of vitamins, minerals, and essential fatty acids. The inclusion of vegetables makes it more palatable, and seasonal varieties usually are added.

OTHER PRODUCTS DERIVED FROM QUINOA

In addition to the food products mentioned in the chapter, many other products are derived from quinoa. These products are obtained by extracting compounds from quinoa and creating value-added products such as protein concentrates and isolates, starches, and bioactive compounds. Quinoa can be used to produce protein concentrate. A more complex process obtains quinoa protein concentrate. The fat-free germ or embryo is to be isolated first. Then, it goes through a high-temperature extraction at pH 11.5 at 50°C. After that, centrifugation, washing, and centrifugation again are done. Solid residue precipitation is performed at pH 4.8 (isoelectric precipitation), and centrifugation is done once more. The solid matter is washed and repeatedly centrifuged, and vacuum dried at 30°C to obtain a protein concentrate with good functional properties and characteristics. The carbohydrate content is of quinoa consists of 54% of small granular starch with a particle size of 0.6–2 µm. The processing of starch significantly improves the digestibility and affects the final product's

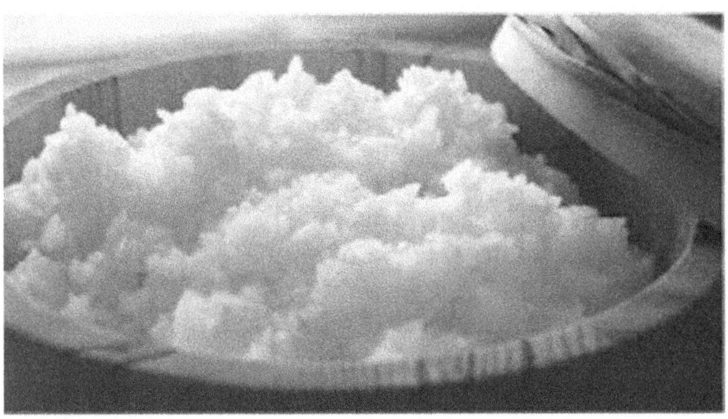

FIGURE 8.4 Quinoa porridge.

binding and organoleptic characteristics. In this respect, compared to the starch content of wheat and barley, quinoa starch shows higher viscosity, higher water retention, expansion capabilities, and higher gelatinization temperatures, resulting in a better performance thickening agent. With such properties, quinoa starch is perfect for producing frozen baby foods. Quinoa may produce edible films and an emulsifier and stabilizing agent based on its high protein and starch content. The incorporation of quinoa in food products has been proven to help extend shelf life and reduce microbial spoilage. The lower degradation rate of starch results in an increase in the shelf life of quinoa-based food products, specifically at the structural and organoleptic levels. Quinoa also provides the microbial preservation of food products, such as inhibiting mold growth when the presence of polyphenolic compounds is considered.

According to a National Library of Medicine study, Amino acids are organic compounds that combine to form proteins. Our body uses various amino acids to make proteins help the body break down food, grow, repair body tissue, and perform many other body functions.

The development of foods rich in amino acids, fibers, minerals, and fatty acids must also be free of antinutritional factors, mainly due to dietary restrictions living with celiac disease. Products made from corn, rice, soybean, tapioca, amaranth seeds, and pseudo cereal such as quinoa can benefit patients with celiac disease. Various products have been developed by using a combination of flours at different levels because the combination of flours improves the nutritional quality and the acceptability of the products. Quinoa seeds have been identified for making soups and desserts, pastries, drinks, and dry snacks.

Following is a brief description of traditional preparations that are made from quinoa in South America.

1. Quinoa soup: Not very thick cooked quinoa with meat or dried meat, tubers, and vegetables.
2. Lawa: A semi-thick 'Mazamorra' (porridge-like preparation) with raw flour, water with lime, and animal fat.
3. P'esque: Quinoa grain cooked with water, without salt, served with either milk or grated cheese according to the availability of these additions.
4. Kispiña: Steamed buns of different shapes and sizes.
5. Tacti o tactacho: Fried buns, a doughnut made with flour and llama fat.
6. Mucuna: Steam-cooked balls made from quinoa flour with seasoning in the center similar to tamales or humitas.
7. Phiri: Roasted and slightly dampened rough quinoa flour.
8. Phisara: Lightly roasted and cooked quinoa grain.
9. Q's: Quinoa chicha, a macerated cold drink.
10. El Ullphu, Ullphi: Cold drink prepared with roasted quinoa flour diluted in water with sugar added to taste.
11. Kaswira de quinua: Flattened bread fried in oil, made with katahui (lime) and white quinoa.
12. Kaswira de Ajara: Flattened bread fried in oil, made with katahui (lime) and black quinoa or Ajara

13. K'api kispiña: Steamed bun, made with quinoa ground in a Kóna and cooked in a clay pot, standard in the feast of all Saints.
14. Turucha quispiña o Polonca: Large steamed pieces of bread, made with katahui and quinoa lightly ground (Chama) in a Kóna and cooked in a clay pot.
15. Mululsito quispiña: Steamed bread, made with katahui and quinoa flour, cooked in a clay pot, smaller than Kispiñas.
16. Quichi quispiña: Steamed and fried bread, made with katahui and quinoa flour, fried in a pan.
17. Juchacha: Andean soup based on ground quinoa and katahui, accompanied by roasted barley flour.
18. Chiwa: Young leaves of quinoa called Lliccha in Quechua and Chiwa in Aymara are used as a vegetable to prepare soups and salads. The leaves are rich in vitamins and minerals, especially calcium, phosphorus, and iron pan.
19. Many international food industry brands are promoting quinoa products under various categories. The future of quinoa products seems very promising as it possess remarkable nutritional properties.

BIBLIOGRAPHY

Al Shehry, G. A. (2016). Use of corn and quinoa flour to produce bakery products for celiac disease. *Adv Environ Biol* 10(12):237–244.

Demir, M. K. and Kilinç, M. (2017). Utilization of quinoa flour in cookie production. *Int Food Res J* 24:2394–2401.

Li, B., Gao, K., Ren, H., and Tang, W. (2018). Molecular mechanisms governing plant responses to high temperatures. *J Integr Plant Biol* 60:757–779.

Li, T., Yang, X., Yu, Y., Si, X., Zhai, X., Zhang, H., Dong, W., Gao, C., and Xu, C. (2018). Domestication of wild tomato is accelerated by genome editing. *Nat Biotechnol* 36:1160–1163.

Liu, J., Wang, R., Liu, W., Zhang, H., Guo, Y., and Wen, R. (2018) Genome-wide characterization of heat-shock protein 70s from *Chenopodium quinoa* and expression analyses of Cqhsp70s in response to drought stress. *Genes* 9.

Pande, M. and Pathak, A. (2009). An overview of Chenopodium album (Bathua sag) chemistry and pharmacological profile. *Journal of Pharmacy and Chemistry* 3(3):79–81.

Poonia, A. and Upadhayay, A. (2015). Chenopodium album Linn: Review of nutritive value and biological properties. *J Food Sci Technol* 52(7):3977–3985.

Prince, S. B. R, Kumar, V., Chandra, S., Kumar, M., and Singh, G. R. (2018). Physicochemical properties of quinoa (Chenopodium quinoa Willd) flakes and corn (Zea mays L) flakes. *Int J Chem Stud* 6(3):1780–1784.

Sharma, V., Chandra, S., Dwivedi, P., and Parturkar, M. (2015). Quinoa (Chenopodium quinoa Willd): A nutritional healthy grain. *Int J Adv Res* 3(9):725–736.

9 Chia Seed Products/ Recipes

Chia seeds have become known as the all-powerful superfood that they are. There is a long list of benefits for these nutrient-packed tiny seeds. Chia seeds are supposed to have a complete set of protein with almost three times more iron than spinach, almost double the amount of potassium than bananas. They are considered a great source of dietary fibers to help digestion. These chia seeds may be tiny, but the word 'chia'itself means 'strength', derived from the Mayan language. Chia seeds may be used in various ways because of their mildly nutty flavor and excellent bite. They may be added to a sweet dish or a savory dish to get an extra energy bump. There are hundreds of ways chia seeds can be incorporated into our diet, and the nutritional profile may be enhanced. Although it is impossible to write and mention all the products and recipes of chia in this chapter, we have tried to put some best combinations and ways to enrich the human diet using chia seeds. It can be included in vegetarian and nonvegetarian diets and is sometimes considered a perfect vegan substitute.

Some of the major food items prepared using chia as the main ingredients are mentioned in this chapter. The nutritive value of the product makes it consider a functional food and also has satiety value. The products from chia are considered excellent appetite suppressing foods so consumed by diet-conscious consumers.

SALMON WITH CHIA

This is a unique recipe in which wild salmon is pan-seared and coated with chia seeds. The wild salmon have hard-to-get eicosapentaenoic acids (EPA), which are mainly found in fatty fishes.

In this dish, fennel is also added rich source of potassium, fiber, folate, and vitamin C. Fresh herbs are also added along with pickled onions.

Its one serving (½ the recipe) provides 410 calories, 31.3 g of fat (4.3 g of saturated fat), 12.1 g of carbs, 3.9 g of fiber, and 30.4 g of protein.

SWEET POTATO CHIA

This is a breakfast recipe that is very rich in potassium due to bananas and sweet potatoes. Potassium is thought to have beneficial effects on sore muscles, which happen after a work out. One banana offers 452 mg of potassium. In comparison, one medium sweet potato adds 716 mg, reported by the USDA.

DOI: 10.1201/9781003080770-9

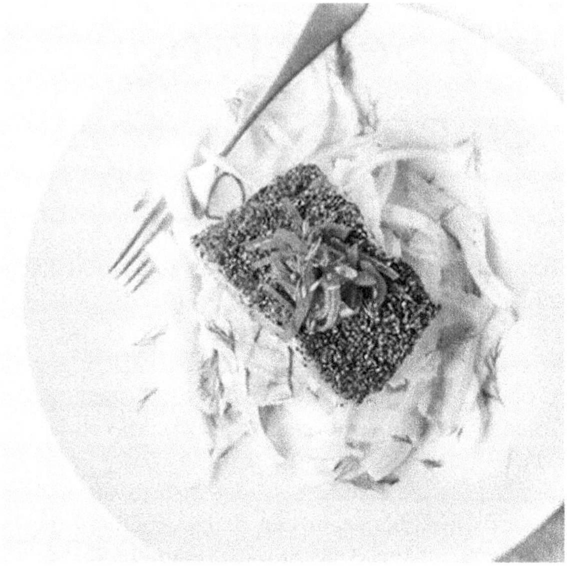

FIGURE 9.1 Salmon with chia.

Moreover, the chia seeds' healthy fats help our body absorb the beta-carotene present in sweet potatoes. The bright color of sweet potatoes is due to the beta-carotene pigment, which also gets converted into vitamin A in the body.

Each sweet potato in this recipe provides 275 calories, 9.8 g of fat (1 g of saturated fat), 44.9 g of carbs, 9.6 g of fiber, and 7.8 g of protein.

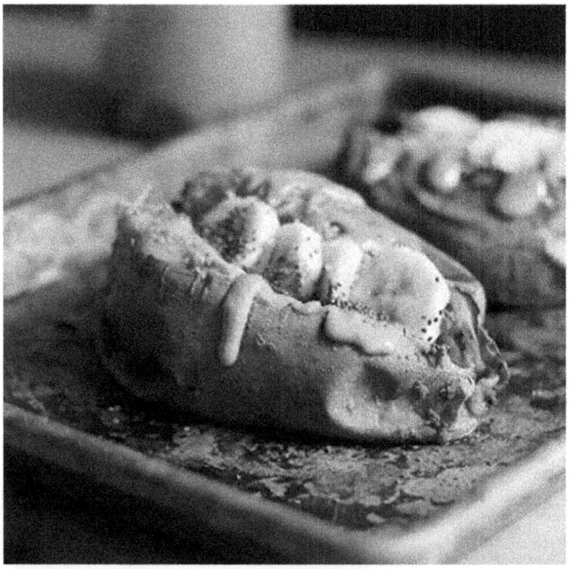

FIGURE 9.2 Sweet potato chia.

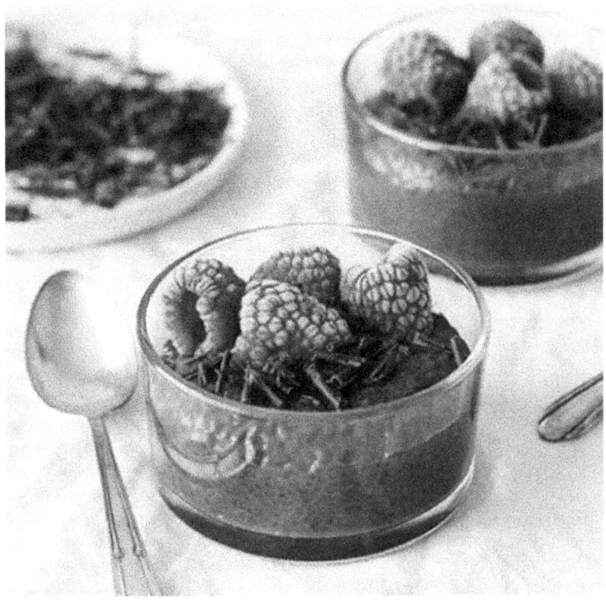

FIGURE 9.3 Chia coco dessert.

CHIA COCO DESSERT

For occasional dessert, the nutrient-rich chocolate chia seed pudding recipe comes as a perfect example. All we need are five simple ingredients such as chia seeds, liquefied cocoa or cacao powder, skimmed milk, maple syrup, and flavor such as vanilla.

The unsweetened cocoa provides nutrients that reduce inflammation, boost HDL cholesterol, reduce high blood pressure, and provide insulin resistance. Nutrients such as flavanols, methylxanthines, and polyphenols are present in cocoa.

It is prepared a few hours before serving as refrigeration is necessary to get a good taste and flavor. Dressing of raspberries, coconut cream, nuts, and whipped cream is also done before consumption.

One serving of the recipe provides 235 calories, 10 g of fat (1 g of saturated fat), 34 g of carbs, 13 g of fiber, and 7 g of protein.

CHIA FRUIT SALAD AND DIP

Chia seeds can add extra nutritional value to our daily favorites, such as salads, fruit punch, boiled/poached eggs, and soups. We may sprinkle them generously over our food to get a boosting effect of omega-3 fatty acids, protein, and fiber. They have a bland flavor that will not impact the taste and bring great texture to the plate.

We may prepare superfood guacamole, hummus, or Greek Tzatziki sauce with chia seeds. Incorporating these tiny chia seeds into our favorite dips will pack a super healthy fruit punch and create a smooth gelatin texture.

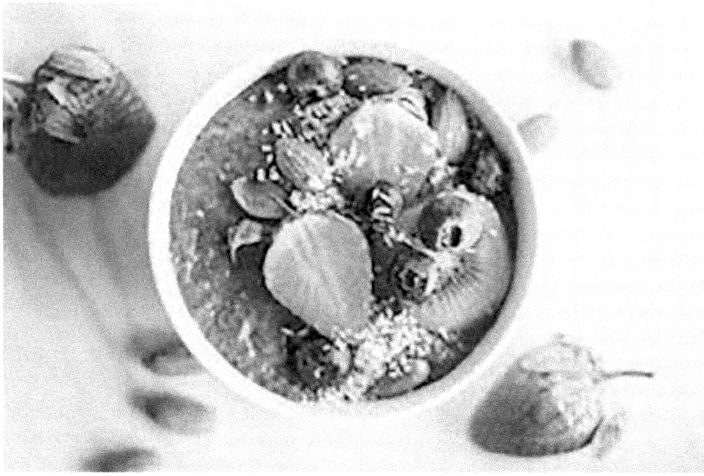

FIGURE 9.4 Chia fruit salad dip.

EGG REPLACED PANCAKES

Chia seeds are among the ways to stick to a vegan diet, as they can create almost the same texture that eggs create. We may prepare one chia seed egg by combining one tablespoon of chia seeds with 3–6 tablespoons of water, and then mixing is done. The mixture is allowed to sit for about 10 minutes, and we can find a perfect egg replacer having the same consistency in bakery products.

CHIA BREAKFAST BARS

Crackers and bars of chia, sesame seeds, pumpkin, and sunflower seeds are very nutritious. These can be prepared by combining about half a cup of each seed and one cup of water and baking as a thin sheet in the oven at 300 degrees for about 30 minutes. For having good flavor and crispiness, the baking step is most crucial. We may add more herbs and spices to bring better taste to chia bars.

CHIA DESSERTS

Desserts are among the favorites of all age groups, and these are hard to resist when craving becomes vital for sweetness. However, healthy desserts are still hard to find. Chia-incorporated desserts may answer all these problems by adding only one or two spoons of chia seeds to the prepared dessert. They will also bring consistency, crispiness, and crunchiness to the foods.

CHIA COVERED MEAT/FISH TENDERS

Chefs always coat meat and fish in starch to make a smooth and whole product appealing. However, instead of using starch, if one tablespoon of chia seeds is used, it will create a crunchy crust. We may also add almond flour or oatmeal flour with

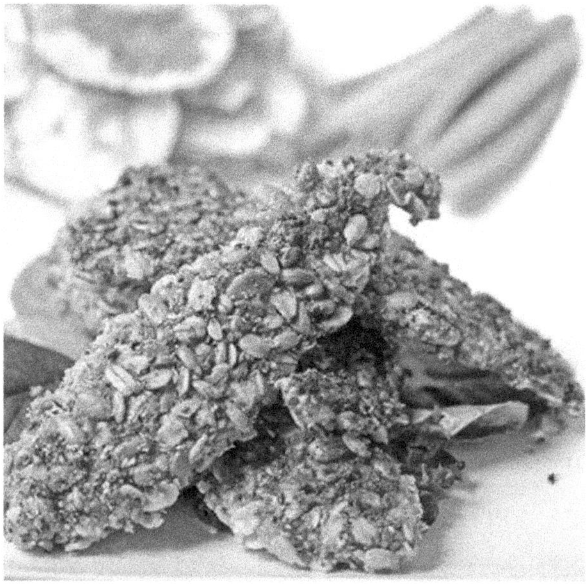

FIGURE 9.5 Meat tenders with chia.

chia seeds resulting in enhanced nutritive value and great color and flavor. Some spices can also be added. The frying process must be avoided, although baking is a better option to prevent nutrient loss.

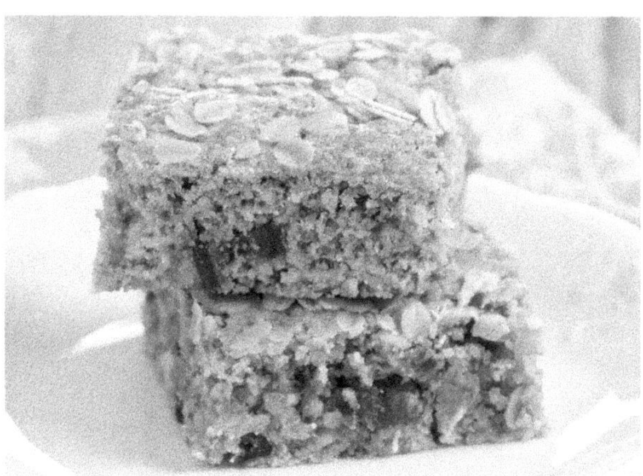

FIGURE 9.6 Breakfast bars.

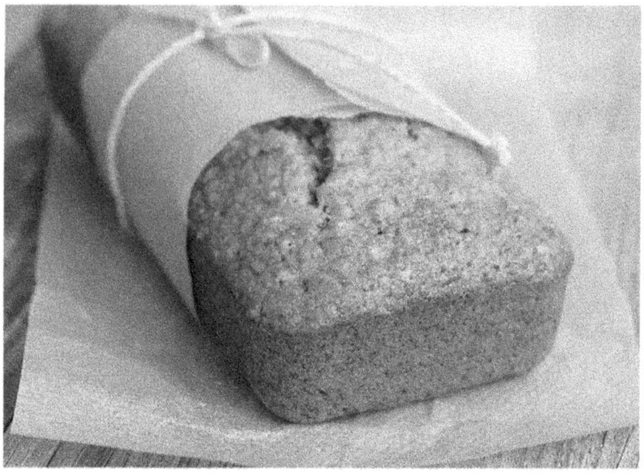

FIGURE 9.7 Chia protein dessert.

CHIA ICE CREAM POPS

For a hot summery day, ice creams are a savior. However, these are packed with refined sugars, artificial colors, and fats. To cover up, we may add berries, oat flakes, coconut milk cream, and chia seeds to ice cream pops to provide a healthy dose of vitamins minerals with good quality fats. They are straightforward to prepare as only blending and freezing are required after preparing the main stuff.

CHIA TORTILLAS

These are made up of chia seeds and are very smooth and light. To prepare these chia tortillas, we combine one and a half cups of whole wheat flour, two tablespoons of flax meal, two tablespoons of chia seeds, one-fourth teaspoon of baking powder, and one tablespoon oil, mainly coconut or olive oil, and some water. Mixing is done and then rolled into a ball-like structure. Then the pan is heated to medium temperature,

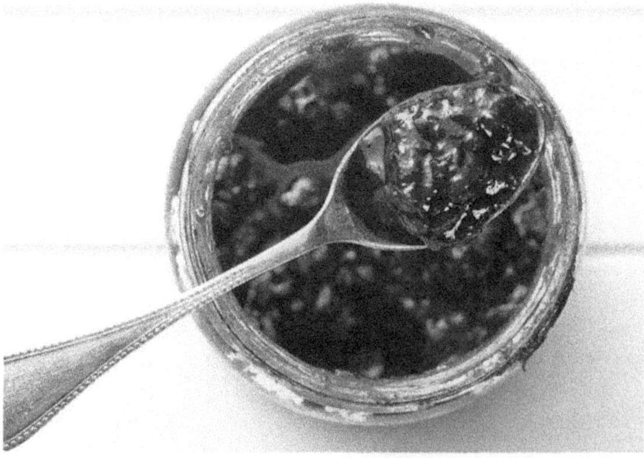

FIGURE 9.8 Chia jam.

and the dough is placed in the pan (without greasing) for a few minutes until light golden brown colored tortillas are prepared. The addition of spices will result in making more flavored and aromatic tortillas.

CHIA TEA AND SMOOTHIES

The addition of chia seeds to tea or smoothy is another good option to enhance the nutritional profile of our hot/iced beverage, imparting a new texture and flavor to it, resulting in many healing benefits for health and improving metabolism.

We may prepare this by combining all ingredients of our preference of fruits and ice depending on the desired texture in a blender. After checking, consistency and addition of more liquid are done if necessary.

CHIA JAM

Fruit jams are all-time favorites of children, and by combing chia seeds, we may create an excellent jam in terms of flavor and taste. Chia seeds make an excellent jelly-like texture, and by simply mashing up chia with fruit pieces, we can get amazing enriched fruit jam. It will result in a more healthy version of the market jam-packed with unhealthy sugars and texturizing agents.

OTHER PRODUCTS

Chia seeds are consumed worldwide, and every country has its unique and unparallel way of preparing delicious dishes. Chia seeds are seen consumed in hundreds of ways by adding in different types of dishes. It can be used as an additional food ingredient, and it is effortless to incorporate these seeds into all forms of food. These are added in puddings, biscuits, cookies, juices, lemonades, frozen desserts, canned products, and many other food products.

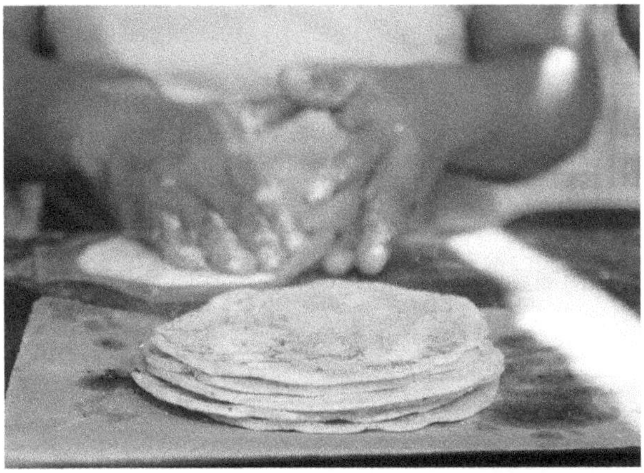

FIGURE 9.9 Chia tortilla.

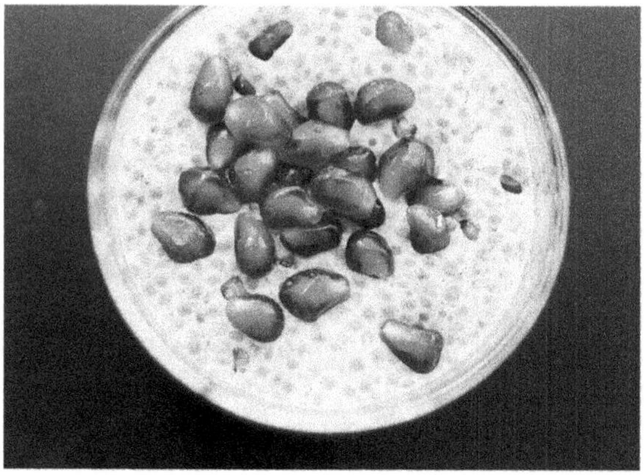

FIGURE 9.10 Chia pudding.

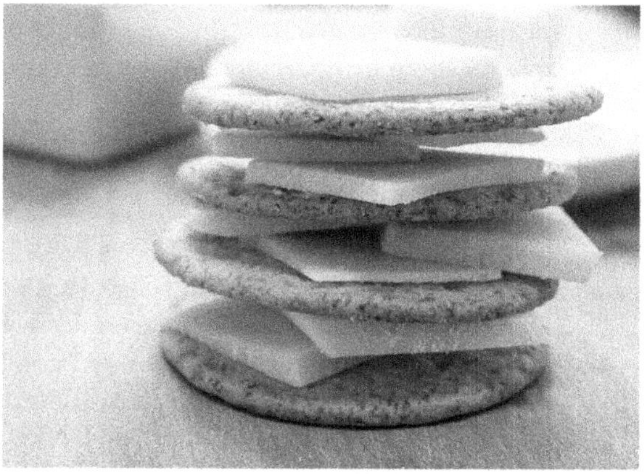

FIGURE 9.11 Chia crunch snack.

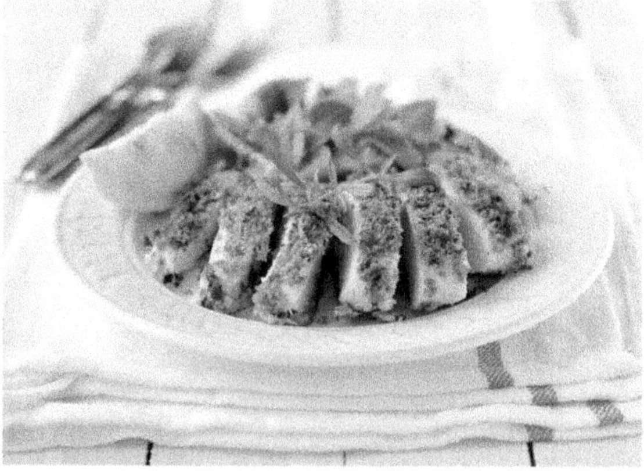

FIGURE 9.12 Chia meat fish crusting.

Keeping in view the nutritional and functional properties of chia seeds, it may be confirmed that chia will be a superfood of the next era.

REFERENCE

Powerful Health Benefits of Turmeric for GERD.... https://drhealthbenefits.com/herbal/herbal-plant/health-benefits-of-turmeric-for-gerd

10 Future Aspects

The market of functional foods has grown exponentially with increasing public health awareness worldwide. The use of nutraceutical or, better says, medicinal food to prevent hypertension, thyroid disorders, diabetes, obesity, and cardiovascular problems is gaining momentum. Seed from *Salvia hispanica* L., more commonly known as chia, is traditional in central and southern America. Currently, widely consumed for various health benefits, it is known for maintaining healthy serum lipid levels. chia contains phenolic acid and omega 3/6, and due to this, various health benefits may be achieved. However, the safety and efficacy of chia seed active ingredients as nutraceutical food or natural product requires validation by more scientific research. Limited *in vivo* and clinical studies on chia seeds' safety aspects and efficacy are available to date.

People are becoming more curious about the properties of chia seeds in recent years. Scientists are getting involved in this material. Various perspectives for the use of chia seeds relate to health and technological aspects. chia seeds can be a part of the new foodstuffs with health-promoting qualities. Seeds of chia are a source of fiber and can also be recommended for diabetes and people with hypercholesterolemia. There are numerous methods and ways for the use of chia in dishes. Chia is considered unique because of its attractive-looking gel-forming characteristic, and the seeds can also be used in flour or whole seeds. Currently, chia seeds are used in many countries as a component of cereal products, e.g., breakfast cereals, rice crisps, wafers, chips. It has been found that the industrial use of chia as a fat or egg substitute in food products does not significantly affect their technological or physical properties.

The future of chia is auspicious as there are many gastronomical recipes for food products having chia as the main component. Although, its industrial application is hindered by the fact that it is still considered a novel food ingredient due to the mentioned legal status of the seed.

Chia seeds incorporated bakery products, yogurt, fruit and vegetable mixes, smoothies, shakes, Ready To Serve beverages, and canned products are used by consumers nowadays. Also, it can be used as an active ingredient in various medicinal foods. We have discussed its nutritional, physical, chemical, and functional properties along with chia products in detail in this book. Looking at its magnificent attributes, we may say that chia is a future crop, and it will be proven as a substitute for the traditional cereal and pulses in many of the products.

QUINOA

As discussed earlier, quinoa is a historical grain believed to have been first domesticated around 5,000 BC. The crop is known for its unique characteristics and has fed the ancient Andean civilization in South America but lost its dominance as a staple

DOI: 10.1201/9781003080770-10

food after the Spanish era started. Quinoa is marvelously nutritious and is often promoted and marketed as a 'superfood'. This super grain is gluten-free and contains essential carbohydrates, fiber, significant vitamins, and minerals essential for human nutrition. The glycemic index of quinoa is much lower than any other cereal crop, so it is beneficial for people with diabetes. Quinoa crops can tolerate a wide range of environmental stress unsuitable for other crops, including salty soils and high altitudes, and withstand a wide range of temperatures.

Even though quinoa grain has multiple benefits and huge agronomic potential, global consumption of quinoa is relatively less than other grains such as cereals like wheat, rice, barley, or corn. Farmers do not prefer its cultivation because it is vulnerable to destruction from rough weather. The plant bears long stalks and small seed heads that make it vulnerable to destruction from inclement weather. Scientists believe that they will manipulate the uncovered genome to produce more significant varieties of grain. By motivating growers to produce shorter and stockier plants that would support larger seed heads, crop production is likely to be much more prominent. The plant produces bitter-tasting seeds that come from one category of chemical compounds named saponins. The saponin removal process is labor-intensive and requires a large quantity of water, making it more costly. The taste and quantity of quinoa yields can be significantly improved by altering recently identified genomes of saponins.

Quinoa's production and marketization are organized according to global trends that heavily affect the market in the forthcoming decade. To visualize that, we need to contextualize quinoa's production in the current global environmental, social, and marketing situation. Important to mention that climatic changes have created disparity amongst various dependent entities such as wildlife, forestry, marine, and humanity. Therefore, the UN has emphasized the change in diet and has been laid to consume a plant-based diet and decrease meat-based products.

When disposable income rises, individuals consume more meat due to cultural norms and marketing for profiteering; therefore, an excellent alternative substitute must be provided to meat if we wish to cope with environmental and health-related needs. Second, and consequently, consumer awareness in the market has seen an increase. The demand for more healthy, eco-friendly, and safer products has also increased. It must be noted that food insecurity is still present alongside this, and often, areas are long exposed to malnutrition and locations, especially in regions where the economy still revolves around agriculture. Lastly, the Euromonitor has mainly highlighted five top trends regarding changing food markets:

1. dairy and gluten-free foods, commonly termed 'free from' foods; considered the most effective in health and wellness. 'Free from' foods alongside plant-based diets are critical factors in abating meat consumption;
2. the rising demand for organic and natural foods, although the definition of organic is debatable and varies across borders;
3. functional foods or value-added products that provide additional benefits to the health of a person in comparison to standard nutritional attributes of a food product,
4. the energy-boosting foods, which maintain longer durations of energy, for instance, paleo and keto diets,

5. paradigm shifts in packaged foods shopping habits lead to subscription meal kits that focus on 'Health and Wellness (HW)', a niche whose growth factor is faster than conventional packaged food. For instance, in the United States, 65% of adults are looking for added minerals and vitamins in their meals.

A further critical aspect related to the debated environmental impacts, which incorporates the challenges to biodiversity, is land use. It includes the increasing area under cultivation, the phenomenon of farmers opting for mono-cultural agriculture, and the replacement of traditional agricultural methods. In detail, regarding the land-use change, Chelleri et al. noted a 'rapid growth in the percentage of plots dedicated to quinoa mono-cropping in 2012 compared with 2010 and 2008' in the communities studied in Tomave municipality, Bolivia. A study conducted in Peru concerning the international quinoa market was analyzed by Bedoya-Perales et al. in three phenomena: displacement, rebound, and cascade. The study noted the extension of land acreage both in traditional and new producing regions. Thus, as yields increase, it can change traditional agricultural methods, may expand the land area and new techniques and technologies. Bedoya-Perales et al. noted the impacts of environmental stress such as loss of genetic biodiversity and 'the emergence of difficult-to-control pests' of the boom related to the cascade effect in traditional quinoa-producing areas region of Puno.

Latorre Farfán, in 2017 analyzed the framework of sustainable production in the area of Majes, Arequipa region, and the study highlighted the need for utilization of the resources more efficiently. Land-use change on the local level is necessary to improve future forecasting and achieve more reliable and sustainable agricultural production.

The world's population is expected to increase from 7.4 billion people in 2015 to 9.8 billion people by 2050. If improvements in the world's current food supply and distribution will not be made, a significant part of the population is expected to experience greater food insecurity. Quinoa is an exceptionally stable and highly nutritious food source. Maybe it can be proven a critical crop for future global food security from a supply perspective and a nutritional one.

The use of pseudocereals such as quinoa and chia may represent a promising area for researchers. Their utilization could improve the intake of macromolecules and phytochemicals beneficial to human health. Quinoa and chia both possess high nutritional characteristics, so they can be promoted as a portion of highly healthy food and super grains of the future. As these grains offer excellent nutritional quality and have a high commercial value, it is thought that more research is needed to increase individuals' awareness of this pseudo-grains nutritional content and consumption. This may help to reveal its nutritional benefits and to investigate its effects on health.

BIBLIOGRAPHY

Chelleri, L., Waters, J., Olazabal, M., and Minucci, G. (2015). Resilience tradeoffs: addressing multiple scales and temporal aspects of urban resilience. *Environ Urban* 27(1):181–198.

Latorre Farfán, J. P. (2017). Is Quinoa Cultivation on the Coastal Desert of Peru Sustainable? A Case Study from MAJES, Arequipa. Master's Thesis, Aarhus University, Aarhus, Denmark.

Index

Note: **Bold** page numbers refer to tables and *italic* page numbers refer to figures.

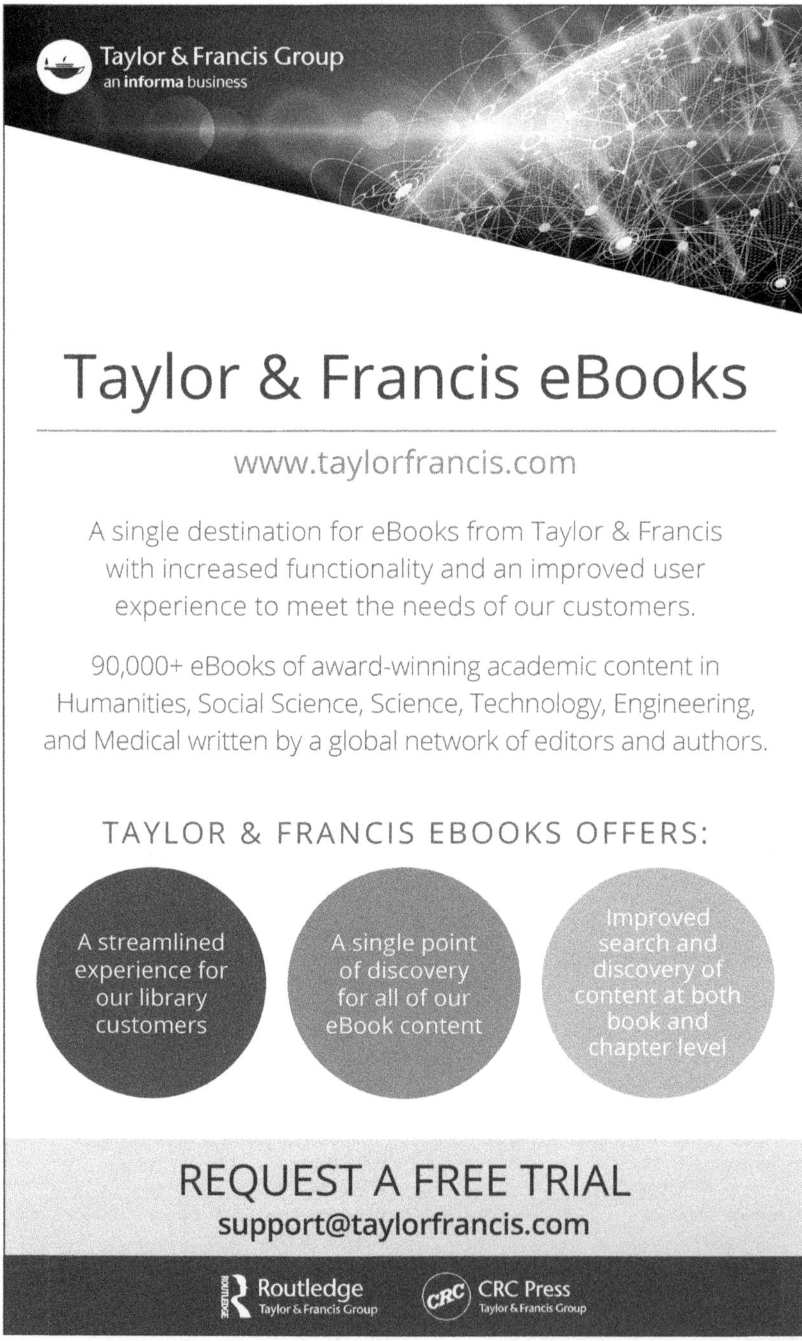

Taylor & Francis Group
an informa business
Taylor & Francis eBooks
www.taylorfrancis.com
A single destination for eBooks from Taylor & Francis with increased functionality and an improved user experience to meet the needs of our customers.
90,000+ eBooks of award-winning academic content in Humanities, Social Science, Science, Technology, Engineering, and Medical written by a global network of editors and authors.
TAYLOR & FRANCIS EBOOKS OFFERS:
A streamlined experience for our library customers
A single point of discovery for all of our eBook content
Improved search and discovery of content at both book and chapter level
REQUEST A FREE TRIAL
support@taylorfrancis.com
Routledge Taylor & Francis Group
CRC Press Taylor & Francis Group

For Product Safety Concerns and Information please contact our EU
representative GPSR@taylorandfrancis.com
Taylor & Francis Verlag GmbH, Kaufingerstraße 24, 80331 München, Germany

www.ingramcontent.com/pod-product-compliance
Ingram Content Group UK Ltd.
Pitfield, Milton Keynes, MK11 3LW, UK
UKHW011019180926
475701UK00004B/831

* 9 7 8 1 0 3 2 2 1 4 6 1 0 *